DIGESTIVE DISEASES - RESEARCH AND CLINICAL DEVELOPMENTS

EOSINOPHILIA

CAUSES, SYMPTOMS AND TREATMENT OPTIONS

Digestive Diseases - Research and Clinical Developments

Additional books in this series can be found on Nova's website under the Series tab.

Additional e-books in this series can be found on Nova's website under the e-book tab.

DIGESTIVE DISEASES - RESEARCH AND CLINICAL DEVELOPMENTS

EOSINOPHILIA

CAUSES, SYMPTOMS AND TREATMENT OPTIONS

ROSANNA FINLAY
EDITOR

New York

For permission to use material from this book please contact us:
Telephone 631-231-7269; Fax 631-231-8175
Web Site: http://www.novapublishers.com

Additional color graphics may be available in the e-book version of this book.

Library of Congress Cataloging-in-Publication Data

ISBN: 978-1-63321-355-5

Published by Nova Science Publishers, Inc. † New York

Contents

Preface

Eosinophilic esophagitis (EoE) is a chronic inflammatory condition characterized clinically by symptoms of esophageal dysfunction and histologically by dense eosinophilic infiltration. Its pathogenesis involves an immune-mediated response to environmental antigenic stimulation. The incidence and prevalence are increasing and EoE has become the most common cause of dysphagia and food impaction in adults. Its management often requires a multi-disciplinary approach as treatment includes specialized diets, anti-eosinophilic medications and esophageal dilation once fibrostensosis has developed. This book discusses the causes, symptoms and treatment options of eosinophilia.

Chapter 1 – Eosinophilic esophagitis (EoE) is a chronic inflammatory condition characterized clinically by symptoms of esophageal dysfunction and histologically by dense eosinophilic infiltration. Its pathogenesis involves an immune-mediated response to allergens. Its management often requires a multi-disciplinary approach with the collaboration of a gastroenterologist, allergist, and nutritionist. Treatment includes specialized diets, anti-eosinophilic medications and esophageal dilation once fibrostensosis has developed. Specialized diets can include anti-allergenic elemental formulation, skin allergy testing directed elimination, or empiric six food elimination diets. With regards to anti-eosinophil medication, the mainstay treatment consists of topical steroids... Esophageal dilation is usually reserved for management of EoE-associated strictures, which are believed to be a result of chronic esophageal inflammation and remodeling. This chapter provides a summary of the three approaches to the management of EoE.

Chapter 2 – Eosinophilic esophagitis (EoE) is an emerging, chronic and immune-driven inflammatory disorder of the esophagus, affecting both children and adults. Clinically, it is characterized by symptoms related to esophageal dysfunction, while histologically it presents with eosinophil predominant inflammation. The prevalence appears to be increasing, particularly in developed countries in parallel with an increase with food allergies. In children the prevalence is estimated to be approximately 1 in 10.000. It has been described as a predominantly male disorder, being at least three-times more frequent in males than in females. The clinical manifestations are diverse in the different age groups. While in infancy, symptoms such as irritability, food refusal, regurgitation and failure to thrive are more common, in school age children symptoms such as nausea, heartburn, dyspepsia and abdominal pain are the more frequent. Only older children and adolescents usually present with adult-like symptoms such as food bolus impaction and dysphagia. A coexistent IgE-mediated food allergy or other allergy driven symptoms such as eczema, rhinitis and asthma are often but not always present. In fact, up to 25% of children with EoE have no evidence of either food or inhalant sensitization. The diagnosis requires fulfillment of clinical, endoscopic and histological criteria. Clinically, it is important to rule out pathologic gastro-esophageal reflux, evidenced by a poor response to 8 weeks of proton-pump inhibitor treatment or a normal 24 hour pH-impedence esophageal monitoring. Endoscopic features include linear furrowing, mucosal fragility, rigid esophageal rings "trachealization", white mucosal plaques and reduced organ caliber, which are typically found along the entire length of the esophagus. Importantly, a macroscopically normal esophageal appearance does not rule out EoE. Histologically, the most commonly accepted definition is based on the evidence of at least 15 eosinophils per high power field (HPF) on esophageal histology at 400-times magnification. Allergic evaluation of patients with EoE mainly relies on skin prick testing (SPT) and atopy patch testing (APT). SPT may be able to guide targeted elimination diets or identify a specific aeroallergen which may also be involved in the pathogenesis of EoE. APT aims to assess cellular response to epicutaneous exposure of food allergens. The treatment of EoE pursues several goals: control of symptoms, correction of complications and prevention of long term sequelae. The two main pillars in the treatment of EoE are food allergen elimination (by means of an elemental or a specific food elimination diet) and/or topical corticosteroids (in the form of topical fluticasone or budesonide). Systemic corticosteroids (prednisolone) are effective but rarely used due to systemic steroid toxicity, particularly in children. Several other medications have been used in the treatment of EoE such as montelukast and biological therapies based on monoclonal antibodies such as mepolizumab and reslizumab. Data on the use of these medications in children are scanty, therefore their use is still limited. In addition to medical treatment, endoscopic food disimpaction and dilatation of strictures is sometimes required. There is paucity of data on both the natural history and optimal long term management of EoE.

Chapter 3 – Eosinophilis are important cells in inflammatory processes, organ and tissue injury and fibrosis. Eosinophilia, resulting from increased bone marrow poiesis and subsequent tissue accumulation, can cause a broad and variegate spectrum of disorders (infectious, connective, allergic, neoplastic and idiopathic disease). In developed countries allergic or atopic disorders are prevailing among paediatric population. A classification of hypereosinophilia based on eosinophilis count has been established: mild form (351-1500/mmc), moderate form (1501-5000/mmc) and severe form (>5000/mmc). An increase in tissue eosinophilia may be seen with or without concomitant peripheral eosinophilia. Clinical presentation and degree of eosinophilia may be very different in relation to the organ which is involved. An higher risk of complications has been described in moderate to severe forms independently from aetiology and is related to tissue and organ infiltration. A detailed medical and familiar history including gastrointestinal, atopic, infective and systemic symptoms should be recorded, including possible recent travel and use of medications. Physical examination should include cardiorespiratory and abdominal evaluation with attention to masses and haepatosplenomegaly and search for dysmorphisms, lymphonodal and articolar involvement and dermatologic lesions (e.g.: rash, signs of haemorragic diathesis). In the clinical approach to a child with eosinophilia first level blood examination (blood cell counts, coagulation profile, haepatic and renal function, inflammatory markers and immunoglobulin) can help in discriminating the possible aetiology and therefore guide the second level examinations (specific allergic tests, immunologic, infectious and onco-haematological work-up). When an underlying cause is not identified idiopathic hypereosinophilia must be considered and at present, a diagnosis of primary eosinophilia mandates a bone marrow examination, karyotype analysis, and molecular studies. The treatment of secondary eosinophilia depends on the aetiology and therefore demands the therapeutic option to a specific setting. In case of idiopathic hypereosinophilia instead, the therapy includes steroids as first line, hydroxyurea, interferon-alpha, chemoterapeuthics and monoclonal antibodies as second line. Allogeneic transplantation offers a viable treatment option for drug-refractory cases.

Chapter 4 – Synovial fluid eosinophilia is defined as the presence of eosinophils, irrespective of quantity, in the synovial fluid. This is a rare, often unexpected, and probably underestimated finding. Secondary and idiopathic forms have been described. Idiopathic forms are those not associated with systemic or rheumatic inflammatory disease or associated with chronic non-inflammatory rheumatic diseases. Idiopathic synovial fluid eosinophilia can be divided into pure or pseudoallergic forms when they occur in patients with an atopic background and/or intensely positive dermographism. Their clinical significance remains incompletely understood. An updated systematic literature review on synovial fluid eosinophilia and eosinophilic arthritis is presented here. Sixty six patients with synovial fluid eosinophilia were identified after search in MEDLINE, EMBASE and Web of Science without publication date restrictions, 31 secondary forms and 35 idiopathic forms, of which 22 were pure idiopathic and 13 were pseudoallergic. Both idiopathic forms are usually monoarthritis of the large joints with a substantial component of joint effusion but few inflammatory signs. Most patients have a benign course with prompt resolution and few relapses. Non-steroidal anti-inflammatory drugs are usually sufficient to control symptoms. Peripheral eosinophilia is a rare association and is not usually severe. Synovial fluid eosinophilia, both secondary and idiopathic, has not been associated with the development of new joint deformities nor has it been described as a chronic form of arthritis.

In: Eosinophilia
Editor: Rosanna Finlay

ISBN: 978-1-63321-355-5

Chapter 1

The Management of Eosinophilic Esophagitis

Dustin M. Albert, M.D. and Fouad J. Moawad, M.D.
Walter Reed National Military Medical Center, Bethesda, MD, US

Abstract

Eosinophilic esophagitis (EoE) is a chronic inflammatory condition characterized clinically by symptoms of esophageal dysfunction and histologically by dense eosinophilic infiltration. Its pathogenesis involves an immune-mediated response to allergens. Its management often requires a multi-disciplinary approach with the collaboration of a gastroenterologist, allergist, and nutritionist. Treatment includes specialized diets, anti-eosinophilic medications and esophageal dilation once fibrostensosis has developed. Specialized diets can include anti-allergenic elemental formulation, skin allergy testing directed elimination, or empiric six food elimination diets. With regards to anti-eosinophil medication, the mainstay treatment consists of topical steroids... Esophageal dilation is usually reserved for management of EoE-associated strictures, which are believed to be a result of chronic esophageal inflammation and remodeling. This chapter provides a summary of the three approaches to the management of EoE.

Introduction

Eosinophilic esophagitis (EoE) is a chronic inflammatory condition characterized clinically by symptoms of esophageal dysfunction and histologically by dense eosinophilic infiltration. [1, 2] Its pathogenesis involves an immune-mediated response to environmental antigenic stimulation which results in an over-expression of Th-2 cytokines. [3] The incidence and prevalence are increasing and EoE has become the most common cause of dysphagia and food impaction in adults. [4, 5] Its management often requires a multi-disciplinary approach as treatment includes anti-eosinophilic medications, specialized diets, and esophageal dilation once fibrostenosis has developed. With regards to anti-eosinophil medication, the mainstay of treatment is topical steroids. Studies have utilized formulations of aerosolized swallowed fluticasone and budesonide. Other anti-eosinophilic medications currently under investigation include anti-IgE and anti-IL-5 monoclonal antibodies.

Specialized diets can include anti-allergenic elemental formulation, skin allergy testing directed elimination, or empiric six food elimination diets. Esophageal dilation is usually reserved for management of EoE-associated strictures, which are believed to be a result of chronic esophageal inflammation and remodeling. Herein, the most current evidence in the management of EoE is reviewed to include the benefits of each approach.

Therapeutic Endpoints

Establishing therapeutic endpoints in EoE is a challenge. It remains unclear whether response should be defined clinically, histologically, or if both must be achieved.

Ideally, a histologic resolution of eosinophilia correlates with a clinical improvement. Certainly, some controlled studies have demonstrated a correlation between symptom improvement and histology, [6, 7, 8, 9] while other studies have actually noted discordance between symptoms and histology. [10, 11, 12] In terms of histologic response, studies have used a range of eosinophil endpoints. These include ≤ 1, [10] ≤ 5, [9]' [13] ≤ 7, [14] and < 15 eos/hpf. [15] The nonspecific symptoms of EoE also complicate the measurement of symptomatic response and the correlation with histologic changes.

Medications

Acid Suppressants

A proton pump inhibitor (PPI) trial is recommended in all patients with suspected EoE. There are three reasons for this. The first reason is that an 8-week course of PPI is necessary to establish the diagnosis of EoE, based on expert recommendations. [1, 2] The second reason is to rule out gastroesophageal reflux disease (GERD) and other causes of esophageal eosinophilia, namely PPI-responsive esophageal eosinophilia (PPI-REE). EoE as PPI-REE are clinically, endoscopically, and histologically indistinguishable without a PPI trial. [16, 17] Furthermore, response to PPI would preclude the need for topical steroids or dietary modification. [4] The third reason is that many EoE patients experience clinical improvement with acid suppression. Several studies have demonstrated clinical response even in the absence of typical reflux symptoms, negative pH testing, and negative endoscopic findings. [18, 19]

Topical Corticosteroids

Topical steroids are first-line therapy for EoE. [2] These medications improve esophageal inflammation through inhibition of pro-inflammatory cytokines. [3] The two steroids commonly prescribed in clinical practice are fluticasone and budesonide. There have been two randomized placebo-controlled trials using fluticasone in the treatment of EoE. In a cohort of 36 children, topical fluticasone administered twice daily at a dosage of 440 mcg for 3 months was associated with histologic improvement in 50% (10/20) of patients. [10] In an adult population, 62% (11/15) of EoE patients achieved histologic response with swallowed fluticasone 880 mcg twice daily for 8 weeks. Response was defined as a greater than 90% decrease in pretreatment eosinophilia. Interestingly, there was no significant clinical improvement when compared to placebo. [11]

Budesonide is the other topical corticosteroid commonly prescribed for the treatment of EoE. Controlled studies exist in children and adults. In one randomized placebo-controlled study in children, oral viscous budesonide was effective in improving symptoms, endoscopic findings, and esophageal eosinophilia in 87% of patients (13/15). [8] In contrast, none who received placebo had response. In adults with EoE, oral budesonide has been shown to induce and maintain histologic response. In one randomized controlled trial, 1 mg of oral budesonide for 15 days was effective in significantly improving symptoms and histology. [7] In a follow-up 50-week study, a subset of patients maintained on low dose (0.5 mg) oral budesonide continued to demonstrate both clinical and histologic response. [9] No study to date has compared the two commonly prescribed topical corticosteroids. However, the delivery method of swallowed budesonide may be preferred to that of aerosolized fluticasone, as a swallowed viscous solution improves mucosal contact time. This was demonstrated in one randomized open label study comparing two variations of budesonide in which oral viscous budesonide was more effective than nebulized budesonide in decreasing esophageal eosinophilia. [20]

The role of systemic steroids is less established in the management of EoE, particularly in adults. In the only randomized controlled trial comparing systemic to swallowed fluticasone in children with EoE, prednisone resulted in a slightly greater histologic improvement. However, clinical improvement was similar. Prednisone was associated with more adverse events to include weight gain and Cushinoid features. [2, 21]

Proper preparation and administration are essential for improved response. For fluticasone, EoE patients are instructed to swallow the medicine, rather than inhale. Budesonide is prepared by mixing aqueous respules with a sugar substitute, honey, or xanthan gum to create a slurry referred to as oral viscous budesonide. With both medications, patients should avoid eating or drinking for 30-60 minutes after administration to reduce the likelihood of early drug clearance. Topical steroid therapy is generally safe with very few side effects reported in the literature. The most common side effect is development of candida esophagitis, which occurs in up to 30% of cases. [2] However, these cases are often asymptomatic and discovered incidentally during follow-up endoscopy. [14] Development of candida appears to be dose dependent. [11]

Biologic Agents and Monoclonal Antibodies

There has been an interest in IL-5 as a potential target for EoE therapy given its role in eosinophil activation. [22] To date, anti-IL-5 treatment is experimental and not clinically available. The two IL-5 antibodies studied, mepolizumab and reslizumab, have demonstrated significant histologic response, but no difference in symptomatic response from placebo. [23, 24, 25] The only randomized placebo controlled study using mepolizumab 750 mg administered one week apart in 11 EoE patients demonstrated a significant decrease in eosinophilia in the treatment group. However, no patient achieved complete histologic response and there was no significant improvement in clinical symptoms. [25] Similarly, infliximab was not effective in inducing histologic or clinical improvement in 3 adults with steroid dependent EoE. [26] Finally, omalizumab, an IgE antibody, was not effective in a case series of two adults. [27]

OC000459 is a selective chemoattractant receptor-homologous molecule on Th-2 cells which decreases eosinophilic inflammation in asthma. [28] In a randomized controlled trial, 26 adult patients with active EoE who were either dependent on or resistant to corticosteroids were treated with OC000459 or placebo twice daily for 8 weeks. Patients in the treatment arm had a modest but significant improvement in histologic measures and significant improvement in clinical measures, the latter of which was evaluated by both patient report and physician global assessment. [29]

Dietary

There are three dietary approaches available for the treatment of EoE. These include elemental diet, targeted elimination diet based on skin prick testing and empiric six-food elimination diet (SFED). Elemental diet involves complete elimination of potential food allergens. This method is highly effective in children with up to 98% of patients experiencing resolution of symptoms and histology within 4 weeks. [30, 31, 32, 33] Despite its efficacy, strict adherence to an elemental diet is costly and challenging since it may require placement of feeding tubes for formula administration. Recently, a study reported findings of an elemental diet in an adult population with EoE. [34] After 2-4 weeks of elemental formula, 72 % (13/18) achieved complete or near complete histologic resolution. Several subjects experienced weight loss and 1/3 of the cohort failed to adhere to the diet. Within 1 week of food reintroduction, EoE recurred in all patients. Although this diet is effective, especially in children, its poor palatability and cost make its long-term use in adults impractical.

The second form of dietary therapy for EoE is targeted elimination diet based on allergy testing using skin prick and patch testing to identify potential triggers. Although this restrictive diet is more practical than an aminoacid based formula diet, it is also less efficacious. [33, 35] In the initial study using this method, 69% (18/26) of children demonstrated a complete response with subsequent studies showing response rates ranging from 55-77% in children.

[36, 37, 38] Data in adults is primarily derived from two studies which demonstrated mixed results. Molina-Infante et al. evaluated 15 patients of which 4 (26%) achieved complete remission, whereas 1 patient achieved clinical remission without histologic remission. [39] In a more recent study done by Wolf et al., symptomatic improvement occurred in 68% (15/22), endoscopic improvement was achieved in 53% (10/22), and 32% (6/22) had <15 eos/hpf after treatment, however the number of adults with <5 eos/hpf were not identified. [40] In another study in adults, skin prick testing predicted only 13% of food triggers and 67% of patients who had a food trigger identified by reintroduction had a negative skin prick test to all foods, questioning its role in management. [41] A recent review evaluated 14 different studies showing that the adult population is under studied, but appears to have a lower response rate compared to children. [42] Further studies are necessary to establish validity and standardization before implementation of this approach.

The third approach to dietary therapy is empiric elimination of the most common food allergens. This is known as the six-food elimination diet (SFED) and includes removal of milk, wheat, soy, nuts, egg, and seafood. The first study using this method demonstrated 94% symptomatic and 74% histologic resolution in children with EoE. The most common triggers of EoE upon reintroduction were egg, soy, milk and wheat. [43] This method has also shown similar efficacy in adults. In a study of 50 adults, 94% had symptomatic improvement and 64% achieved histologic remission (<5 eos/hpf). After food was reintroduced, wheat and milk were the most commonly identified allergens. [40] Importantly, there is data supporting long-term remission using this approach. In a study of 67 patients, 37 (55%) achieved a complete histologic response (<5 eos/hpf) and 12 (18%) had a partial histologic response (6-14 eos/hpf). [44] One-year follow-up data was available for 25 patients who successfully continued to avoid the offending foods, all of whom remained asymptomatic and in histologic remission. Fifteen patients completed treatment for 2 years and 4 were able to maintain it for 3 years. All patients remained asymptomatic and were in histological remission without the need for drug treatment. The combined efficacy of SFED between children and adults is 72.1%. [42]

Dilation

Esophageal remodeling is a phenomenon which occurs in long-standing and untreated EoE. Consequently, fibrostenosis develops. [45, 46] On endoscopy, this appears as fixed fibrotic rings (trachealization), a diffusely narrow esophagus or a dominant stricture. Although esophageal dilation does not address the underlying pathophysiology of EoE, it is probably the only effective method to treat strictures, especially when fibrosis has developed. Early studies and case series cautioned against dilation due to high rate of complications, including hemorrhage and perforation. [47, 48, 49, 50, 51, 52, 53] However, larger studies to include a meta-analysis have demonstrated safety and efficacy of dilation in the management of esophageal strictures. [54, 55, 56, 57, 58] The most recent guidelines recommend that dilation be used in symptomatic patients with strictures that persist despite medical or dietary therapy. [2]

Technique

Three methods have been described in the literature: bougie dilation with a Maloney, wire-guided with a Savary, or through-the-scope (TTS) hydrostatic balloon dilation. There are no data to support one technique over the other and these techniques are based on the experience and preference of the endoscopist. Balloon dilation has the theoretical advantage of decreased shear stress injury produced by bougie dilation, the ability to determine esophageal caliber, directly visualize the dilation, allow for inspection of esophageal mucosa between dilations without the need to reintroduce the endoscope, and stopping once a mucosal tear is noted. [2, 4] Bougies, on the other hand, offer the ability to dilate the entire esophagus with one pass, the ability to dilate multiple and long strictures as in a diffusely narrowed esophagus, can provide a tactile sensation of resistance to the endoscopist, and are less expensive. [2, 4] There is no evidence that one technique is safer than the other in patients with EoE. [2]

Regardless of technique, a conservative approach is recommended to reduce the risk of complications. Endoscopists should start with a balloon diameter just smaller than the diameter of the stricture. Two to three dilation sessions separated by 2-3 weeks are typically required when the initial esophageal diameter is 9 mm or less. [59] If a mucosal disruption occurs, no further dilation should be performed during that session. [2] Of note, the extent and depth of mucosal tears does not correlate with chest pain, need for narcotics, or hospitalization. [59] Other than representing a successful dilation, there is limited data to suggest mucosal tears have any other clinical implications.

Efficacy

Dilation for treatment in EoE was first described in 2001 by Morrow et al. [60] In this retrospective study, 19 adults with esophageal stenosis underwent dilation with Savary dilators to achieve an esophageal diameter of 14-15mm. At 19 months, 94% (15/16) reported overall improvements in swallowing. Using a dysphagia scale (0 = no dysphagia, 1 = <once/month, 2 = several times/month, 3 = several times/week, 4 = daily, not every meal and 5 = every meal), the average score improved from 4 to 1.2. A systematic review published by Bohm and Richter found that 92% of patients treated by esophageal dilation had improvement in dysphagia symptoms for up to 1-2 years. [59] In a meta-analysis limited to cohort studies of EoE patients undergoing dilations within a defined time frame, clinical improvement was seen in 75% of patients undergoing dilation. [54]

The largest study to date included a retrospective review of 207 adult EoE patients divided into two cohorts. [61] The first study included 63 patients treated only with dilation and the second study was comprised of 144 patients treated with dilation who were simultaneously receiving pharmacologic therapy. In cohort one, 46 patients were dilated with Savary bougies and 17 by TTS balloons. A median of 2 dilation sessions occurred and an average increase of bougie diameter from 11 to 16 mm. After dilation, 45% had complete resolution of dysphagia and 50% had only minor swallowing difficulties. Notably, 67% of patients reported an improvement of dysphagia lasting >12 months and 41% lasting >24 months. Long-term follow-up data was not available for patients in cohort 2, but patients initially responded similar to those in cohort 1. [59] Notably, 74% of patients experienced retrosternal pain following dilation, described as moderate in 21% and severe in 17%. There were however no perforations, hospitalizations, or bleeding. Importantly, this is the only study that addressed the patients' tolerability and acceptance of undergoing dilation (n = 42). Forty-four percent did not find it cumbersome at all, 36% found it a little cumbersome, and 19% found it very cumbersome. However, all patients questioned thought dilation was acceptable and if indicated, would repeat dilation. Other large studies reported similar clinical efficacy. [56, 57, 58]

Safety

The esophageal wall in EoE has reduced elasticity and is fragile making it susceptible to mucosal tears. Although this has been reported as a complication in several studies, the development of mucosal tears is an intended outcome. [62] The greatest concern of dilation is esophageal perforation which is fortunately rare. In two systematic reviews, the perforation rate was 0.3%, nearly similar to that quoted for dilation in non-EoE patients. [2, 4, 59, 63] Major bleeding, defined as requiring endoscopic hemostasis or a blood transfusion, is rare with only 1 patient reported to date. [2] Notably no deaths resulted from dilation and most perforations were managed non-operatively. [4, 59] The most common risk is post dilation chest pain, which was reported in 74% of 42 patients questioned in one of the largest studies of esophageal dilation. [61] The pain persists at most for several days and responds well to reassurance and analgesics. [59]

Conclusion

The current management strategy of EoE is based on the 3 D's: drugs, diet, and dilation. While only anti-eosinophilic medications and dietary treatment may improve symptoms and histology, dilation is effective in improving symptoms associated with fibrostenotic strictures. Given its complex pathogenesis which remains incompletely understood, a multi-disciplinary approach to the treatment of EoE is recommended. Collaboration between a gastroenterologist, allergist, pathologist and nutritionist will give patients the best possible outcomes.

References

[1] Liacouras CA, Furuta GT, Hirano I, et al. Eosinophilic esophagitis: updated consensus recommendations for children and adults. *J. Allergy Clin. Immunol.* 2011; 128:3-20 e6; quiz 21-2.

[2] Dellon ES, Gonsalves N, Hirano I, et al. ACG clinical guideline: Evidenced based approach to the diagnosis and management of esophageal eosinophilia and eosinophilic esophagitis (EoE). *Am. J. Gastroenterol.* 2013; 108:679-92; quiz 693.
[3] Greenhawt M, Aceves S, Spergel J, Rothenberg M. The Management of Eosinophilic Esophagitis. *J. Allergy Clin. Immunol. Pract.* 2013; 1:332-340.
[4] Dellon ES. Diagnosis and management of eosinophilic esophagitis. *Clin. Gastroenterol. Hepatol.* 2012; 10: 1066-78.
[5] Hruz P. Epidemiology of eosinophilic esophagitis. *Digestive Disease* 2014; 32:40-7.
[6] Aceves SS, Newbury RO, Dohil MA, et al. A symptom scoring tool for identifying pediatric patients with eosinophilic esophagitis and correlating symptoms with inflammation. *Ann. Allergy Asthma Immunol.* 2009; 103:401-6.
[7] Straumann A, Conus S, Degen L, et al. Budesonide is effective in adolescent and adult patients with active eosinophilic esophagitis. *Gastroenterology* 2010; 139: 1526-37, 1537 e1.
[8] Dohil R, Newbury R, Fox L, et al. Oral viscous budesonide is effective in children with eosinophilic esophagitis in a randomized, placebo-controlled trial. *Gastroenterology* 2010; 139:418-29.
[9] Straumann A, Conus S, Degen L, et al. Long-term budesonide maintenance treatment is partially effective for patients with eosinophilic esophagitis. *Clin. Gastroenterol. Hepatol.* 2011; 9:400-409.
[10] Konikoff MR, Noel RJ, Blanchard C, et al. A randomized, double-blind, placebo-controlled trial of fluticasone propionate for pediatric eosinophilic esophagitis. *Gastroenterology* 2006; 131: 1381-91.
[11] Alexander JA, Jung KW, Arora AS, et al. Swallowed fluticasone improves histologic but not symptomatic response of adults with eosinophilic esophagitis. *Clin. Gastroenterol. Hepatol.* 2012; 10:742-749 e1.
[12] Pentiuk S, Putnam PE, Collins MH, et al. Dissociation between symptoms and histological severity in pediatric eosinophilic esophagitis. *J. Pediatr. Gastroenterol. Nutr.* 2009; 48:152-60.
[13] Peterson KA, Thomas KL, Hilden K, et al. Comparison of esomeprazole to aerosolized, swallowed fluticasone for eosinophilic esophagitis. *Dig. Dis. Sci.* 2010; 55:1313-9.

[14] Aceves SS, Bastian JF, Newbury RO, et al. Oral viscous budesonide: a potential new therapy for eosinophilic esophagitis in children. *Am. J. Gastroenterol.* 2007; 102:2271-9; quiz 2280.
[15] Vazquez-Elizondo G, Ngamruengphong S, Khrisna M, et al. The outcome of patients with oesophageal eosinophilic infiltration after an eight-week trial of a proton pump inhibitor. *Aliment Pharmacol. Ther.* 2013; 38:1312-9.
[16] Moawad FJ, Safroneeva E, Ally MR, et al. Eosinophilic oesophagitis and proton pump inbhibitor-responsive oesophageal eosinophilia have similar clinical, endoscopic and histological findings. *Aliment Pharmacol. Ther.* 2014;In press.
[17] Dellon ES, Speck O, Woodward K, et al. Clinical and endoscopic characteristics do not reliably differentiate PPI-responsive esophageal eosinophilia and eosinophilic esophagitis in patients undergoing upper endoscopy: a prospective cohort study. *Am. J. Gastroenterol.* 2013; Dec; 108(12): 1854-60.
[18] Moawad FJ, Veerappan GR, Dias JA, et al. Randomized controlled trial comparing aerosolized swallowed fluticasone to esomeprazole for esophageal eosinophilia. *Am. J. Gastroenterol*. 2013; 108:366-72.
[19] Molina-Infante J, Ferrando-Lamana L, Ripoll C, et al. Esophageal eosinophilic infiltration responds to proton pump inhibition in most adults. *Clin. Gastroenterol. Hepatol.* 2011; 9:110-7.
[20] Dellon ES, Sheikh A, Speck O, et al. Viscous topical is more effective than nebulized steroid therapy for patients with eosinophilic esophagitis. *Gastroenterology* 2012; 143:321-4 e1.
[21] Schaefer ET, Fitzgerald JF, Molleston JP, et al. Comparison of oral prednisone and topical fluticasone in the treatment of eosinophilic esophagitis: a randomized trial in children. *Clin. Gastroenterol. Hepatol.* 2008; 6:165-73.
[22] Rothenberg ME. Biology and treatment of eosinophilic esophagitis. *Gastroenterology* 2009; 137:1238-49.
[23] Spergel JM, Rothenberg ME, Collins MH, et al. Reslizumab in children and adolescents with eosinophilic esophagitis: results of a double-blind, randomized, placebo-controlled trial. *J. Allergy Clin. Immunol.* 2012; 129: 456-63, 463 e1-3.
[24] Assa'ad AH, Gupta SK, Collins MH, et al. An antibody against IL-5 reduces numbers of esophageal intraepithelial eosinophils in children with eosinophilic esophagitis. *Gastroenterology* 2011; 141:1593-604.

[25] Straumann A, Conus S, Grzonka P, et al. Anti-interleukin-5 antibody treatment (mepolizumab) in active eosinophilic oesophagitis: a randomised, placebo-controlled, double-blind trial. *Gut.* 2010; 59:21-30.

[26] Straumann A, Bussmann C, Conus S, et al. Anti-TNF-alpha (infliximab) therapy for severe adult eosinophilic esophagitis. *J. Allergy Clin. Immunol.* 2008; 122:425-7.

[27] Rocha R, Vitor AB, Trindade E, et al. Omalizumab in the treatment of eosinophilic esophagitis and food allergy. *Eur. J. Pediatr.* 2011; 170: 1471-4.

[28] Horak F, Zieglmayer P, Zieglmayer R, et al. The CRTH2 antagonist OC000459 reduces nasal and ocular symptoms in allergic subjects exposed to grass pollen, a randomized, placebo-controlled, double blind trial. *Allergy* 2012; 67:1572-9.

[29] Straumann A, Hoesli S, Bussmann C, et al. Anti-eosinophil activity and clinical efficacy of the CRTH2 antagonist OC000459 in eosinophilic esophagitis. *Allergy* 2013; 68:375-85.

[30] Liacouras CA, Spergel JM, Ruchelli E, et al. Eosinophilic esophagitis: a 10-year experience in 381 children. *Clin. Gastroenterol. Hepatol.* 2005; 3:1198-206.

[31] Kelly KJ, Lazenby AJ, Rowe PC, et al. Eosinophilic esophagitis attributed to gastroesophageal reflux: improvement with an amino acid-based formula. *Gastroenterology* 1995; 109:1503-12.

[32] Markowitz JE, Spergel JM, Ruchelli E, et al. Elemental diet is an effective treatment for eosinophilic esophagitis in children and adolescents. *Am. J. Gastroenterol.* 2003; 98:777-82.

[33] Henderson CJ, Abonia JP, King EC, et al. Comparative dietary therapy effectiveness in remission of pediatric eosinophilic esophagitis. *J. Allergy Clin. Immunol.* 2012; 129:1570-8.

[34] Peterson KA, Byrne KR, Vinson LA, et al. Elemental diet induces histologic response in adult eosinophilic esophagitis. *Am. J. Gastroenterol.* 2013; 108:759-66.

[35] Spergel JM, Brown-Whitehorn TF, Cianferoni A, et al. Identification of causative foods in children with eosinophilic esophagitis treated with an elimination diet. *J. Allergy Clin. Immunol.* 2012; 130:461-7 e5.

[36] Spergel JM, Beausoleil JL, Mascarenhas M, Liacouras CA. The use of skin prick tests and patch tests to identify causative foods in eosinophilic esophagitis. *J. Allergy ClinImmunol.* 2002; 109:363-368.

[37] Liacouras CA, Spergel JM, Ruchelli E, et al. Eosinophilic esophagitis: a 10-year experience in 381 children. *Clin. Gastroenterol. Hepatol.* 2005; 3:1198-1206.

[38] Spergel JM, Andrews T, Brown-Whitehorn TF, et al.Treatment of eosinophilic esophagitis with specific food elimination diet directed by a combination of skin prick and patch tests. *Ann. Allergy Asthma Immunol.* 2005; 95:336-343.

[39] Molina-Infante J, Martin-Noguerol E, Alvarado-Arenas M, et al. Selective elimination diet based on skin testing has suboptimal efficacy for adult eosinophilic esophagitis. *J. Allergy Clin. Immunol.* 2012; 130: 1200-1202.

[40] Wolf W, Jerath M, Sperry SL, et al. Dietary Elimination Therapy Is an Effective Option for Adults With Eosinophilic Esophagitis. *Clin. Gastroenterol. Hepatol.* 2014; In Press.

[41] Gonsalves N, Yang GY, Doerfler B, et al. Elimination diet effectively treats eosinophilic esophagitis in adults; food reintroduction identifies causative factors. *Gastroenterology* 2012; 142:1451-9.

[42] Arias A, Gonzalez-Cervera J, Tenias JM, Lucendo AJ. Efficacy of dietary interventions for inducing histologic remission in patients with eosinophilic esophagitis: A systemic review and meta-analysis. *Gastroenterology* 2014; In press.

[43] Kagalwalla AF, Sentongo TA, Ritz S, et al. Effect of six-food elimination diet on clinical and histologic outcomes in eosinophilic esophagitis.*Clin. Gastroenterol. Hepatol.* 2006; 4:1097-102.

[44] Lucendo A, Arias A, Gonzalez-Cervera J, et al. Empiric 6-food elimination diet induced and maintained prolonged remission in patients with adult eosinophilic esophagitis: A prospective study on the food cause of the disease. *J. Allergy ClinImmunol.* 2013; 131:797-804.

[45] Schoepfer AM, Safroneeva E, Bussmann C, et al. Delay in diagnosis of eosinophilic esophagitis increases risk for stricture formation in a time-dependent manner. *Gastroenterology* 2013; 145:1230-6.

[46] Dellon ES, Kim HP, Sperry SL, et al. A phenotypic analysis shows that eosinophilic esophagitis is a progressive fibrostenotic disease. *Gastrointestinal. Endoscopy* 2014; 79:577-85.

[47] Shim LS, Grehan M.Education and Imaging. Gastrointestinal: oesophageal perforation during endoscopy for food impaction in eosinophilicoesophagitis. *J. Gastroenterology and Hepatology* 2010; 25: 428.

[48] Vasilopoulos S, Murphy P, Auerbach A, et al. The small-caliber esophagus: an unappreciated cause of dysphagia for solids in patients with eosinophilic esophagitis. *Gastrointest. Endosc*. 2002; 55:99-106.

[49] Cohen MS, Kaufman A, DiMarino AJ, Cohen S. Eosinophilic esophagitis presenting as spontaneous esophageal rupture (Boerhaave's syndrome). *Clin. Gastroenterol. Hepatol*. 2007; 5:A24.

[50] Croese J, Fairley SK, Masson JW, et al. Clinical and endoscopic features of eosinophilic esophagitis in adults. *Gastrointest. Endosc.* 2003; 58: 516-22.

[51] Kaplan M, Mutlu EA, Jakate S, et al. Endoscopy in eosinophilic esophagitis: "feline" esophagus and perforation risk. *Clin. Gastroenterol. Hepatol.* 2003; 1:433-7.

[52] Eisenbach C, Merle U, Schirmacher P, et al. Perforation of the esophagus after dilation treatment for dysphagia in a patient with eosinophilic esophagitis. *Endoscopy* 2006; 38Suppl 2:E43-4.

[53] Sgouros SN, Bergele C, Mantides A. Eosinophilic esophagitis in adults: a systematic review. *Eur. J. Gastroenterol. Hepatol.* 2006; 18:211-7.

[54] Moawad FJ, Cheatham JG, DeZee KJ. Meta-analysis: the safety and efficacy of dilation in eosinophilicoesophagitis. *Aliment Pharmacol. Ther.* 2013; 38:713-20.

[55] Schoepfer AM, Gonsalves N, Bussmann C, et al. Esophageal dilation in eosinophilic esophagitis: effectiveness, safety, and impact on the underlying inflammation. *Am. J. Gastroeterol*. 2010; 105:1062-70.

[56] Dellon ES, Gibbs WB, Rubinas TC, et al. Esophageal dilation in eosinophilic esophagitis: safety and predictors of clinical response and complications. *Gastrointest. Endosc.* 2010; 71:706-12.

[57] Ally MR, Dias J, Veerappan GR, et al. Safety of dilation in adults with eosinophilic esophagitis. *Disease of Esophagus* 2013; 26:241-5.

[58] Jung KW, Gundersen N, Kopacova J, et al. Occurrence of and risk factors for complications after endoscopic dilation in eosinophilic esophagitis. *Gastrointest. Endosc*. 2011; 73:15-21.

[59] Bohm M, Richter J. Review article: oesophageal dilation in adults with eosinophilicoesophagitis. *Alimient. Pharmacol. Ther.* 2011; 33:748-757.

[60] Morrow JB, Vargo JJ, Goldblum JR, Richter JE. The ringed esophagus: histological features of GORD. *Am. J. Gastroenterol*. 2001; 96:984-9.

[61] Schoepfer AM, Gonsalves N, Bussmann C, et al. Esophageal dilation in eosinophilic esophagitis: effectiveness, safety, and impact on the underlying inflammation. *Am. J. Gastroenterol*. 2010; 105:1062-70.

[62] Straumann A, Rossi L, Simon HU, et al. Fragility of the esophageal mucosa: a pathognomonic endoscopic sign of primary eosinophilic esophagitis? *Gastrointest. Endosc*. 2003; 57:407-12.

[63] Jacobs JW Jr, Spechler SJ. A systemic review of the risk of perforation during esophageal dilation for patients with eosinophilic esophagitis. *Dig. Dis. Sci.* 2010; 55: 1512-1515.

In: Eosinophilia
Editor: Rosanna Finlay
ISBN: 978-1-63321-355-5

Chapter 2

Eosinophilic Esophagitis in Children

Chiara Mameli M.D., Dario Dilillo M.D., Francesca Penagini M.D., Giulia Ramponi M.D., Matteo Torcoletti M.D. and Gian Vincenzo Zuccotti M.D.
Department of Pediatrics, L. Sacco Hospital, University of Milan, Italy

Abstract

Eosinophilic esophagitis (EoE) is an emerging, chronic and immune-driven inflammatory disorder of the esophagus, affecting both children and adults. Clinically, it is characterized by symptoms related to esophageal dysfunction, while histologically it presents with eosinophil predominant inflammation. The prevalence appears to be increasing, particularly in developed countries in parallel with an increase with food allergies. In children the prevalence is estimated to be approximately 1 in 10.000. It has been described as a predominantly male disorder, being at least three-times more frequent in males than in females. The clinical manifestations are diverse in the different age groups. While in infancy, symptoms such as irritability, food refusal, regurgitation and failure to thrive are more common, in school age children symptoms such as nausea, heartburn, dyspepsia and abdominal pain are the more frequent. Only older children and adolescents usually present with adult-like symptoms such as food bolus impaction and dysphagia. A coexistent IgE-mediated food allergy or other allergy driven symptoms such as eczema, rhinitis and asthma are often but not always present. In fact, up to 25% of children with EoE have no evidence of either food or inhalant sensitization. The diagnosis requires fulfillment of clinical, endoscopic and histological criteria. Clinically, it is important to rule out pathologic gastro-esophageal reflux, evidenced by a poor response to 8 weeks of proton-pump inhibitor treatment or a normal 24 hour pH-impedence esophageal monitoring. Endoscopic features include linear furrowing, mucosal fragility, rigid esophageal rings "trachealization", white mucosal plaques and reduced organ caliber, which are typically found along the entire length of the esophagus. Importantly, a macroscopically normal esophageal appearance does not rule out EoE. Histologically, the most commonly accepted definition is based on the evidence of at least 15 eosinophils per high power field (HPF) on esophageal histology at 400-times magnification. Allergic evaluation of patients with EoE mainly relies on skin prick testing (SPT) and atopy patch testing (APT). SPT may be able to guide targeted elimination diets or identify a specific aeroallergen which may also be involved in the pathogenesis of EoE. APT aims to assess cellular response to epicutaneous exposure of food allergens. The treatment of EoE pursues several goals: control of symptoms, correction of complications and prevention of long term sequelae. The two main pillars in the treatment of EoE are food allergen elimination (by means of an elemental or a specific food elimination diet) and/or topical corticosteroids (in the form of topical fluticasone or budesonide). Systemic corticosteroids (prednisolone) are effective but rarely used due to systemic steroid toxicity, particularly in children. Several other medications have been used in the treatment of EoE such as montelukast and biological therapies based on monoclonal antibodies such as mepolizumab and reslizumab. Data on the use of these medications in children are scanty, therefore their use is still limited. In addition to medical treatment, endoscopic food disimpaction and dilatation of strictures is sometimes required. There is paucity of data on both the natural history and optimal long term management of EoE.

Introduction and Epidemiology

Eosinophilic Esophagitis (EoE) is a chronic immune-mediated esophageal disease characterized histologically by eosinophil-predominant inflammation and clinically by symptoms of esophageal dysfunction [1,2]. Since EoE has been recognized as a clinicopathologic entity in both children and adults only in the recent years, the prevalence and incidence worldwide are difficult to estimate because of the scarcity of large database. Dellon et al. have established a prevalence of 56,7/100.000 persons in the United States, including the pediatric population as well [3]. A recent study conducted by Noel et al. between the years 2000 and 2003 reported an annual incidence of EoE in Ohio, of 1/10.000, leading to an estimated prevalence of 4/10.000 children by the end of 2003 [4].

It is not clear whether childhood EoE is increasing in incidence, and if so, to what extent. A study conducted by van Rhijn et al. checked through a nationwide registry the pathology reports in the Netherlands from 1996 through 2010 and classified according to the diagnosis made by the pathologist [5]. The incidence of EoE increased from 0.01/10.000 people in 1996 to 1.31/10.000 people in 2010. Nevertheless, these results are biased by the increased awareness and knowledge on EoE from 2000 onwards, thus the reported increase in incidence must be interpreted with caution.

EoE affects both genders with a male-to-female ratio of 3:1 and all age groups, with a peak incidence in childhood and during the third-fourth decades of life [1]. Both adult and pediatric patients commonly present with a positive history for food allergies, asthma, eczema and chronic rhinitis. There is a high prevalence of IgE and non-IgE mediated food allergy in pediatric patients with EoE. However, up to 25% of children with EoE have no evidence of either food or inhalant sensitization. All ethnic groups are affected, with a predominance in the Caucasian population. A possible geographical variation has been suggested, with an increased frequency in the urban areas.

Immunopathogenesis

The pathogenesis of EoE appears to be immune-mediated, characterized by a predominantly T-helper-2 (Th2) lymphocyte driven disorder with an increase in mucosal eosinophils, mast cells and basophils. The inflammatory response is thought to be triggered by either food or aeroallergen antigens which would activate the production of proinflammatory cytokines leading to eosinophil recruitment in esophageal mucosa [6]. Indeed, there is evidence in both humans and experimental models that also inhaled aeroallergens (including pollens and molds) can induce esophageal eosinophilia [7]. The migration of eosinophils into the esophagus is under the control of three crucial effector molecules: IL-5, IL-13 and Eotaxin-3.

Eotaxin-3, a powerful chemokine triggered by IL-13, is thought to play an important role in pathogenesis of the eosinophil infiltrate, as it has been found to be up regulated in the mucosa of EoE affected patients. Eotaxin-3 would stimulate the recruitment eosinophils in the esophageal mucosa. The eosinophils, in turn, would secrete proinflammatory mediators, which cause local tissue damage and recruit mast cells and fibroblasts, maintaining subepithelial inflammation and remodeling ultimately leading to fibrosis [6].

Basal cell proliferation is a key histological feature in patients with EoE. Subepithelial remodeling and deposition of collagen has been demonstrated in patients with EoE and may contribute to dysphagia. Eosinophils may also directly disrupt the integrity of submucosal neuronal networks and promote lower esophageal sphincter and peristalstic dysfunction.

Genetics

Numerous studies have suggested EoE's strong genetic inheritability [8, 9]. Indeed, 6.8% of patients with EoE have at least 1 family member suffering from the same disease [10]. Familial clusters of EoE have been described but the exact susceptibility loci for familial and sporadic EoE require further clarification. The two EoE subtypes, sporadic and familial, have been compared for clinical, endoscopic and pathological features and global esophageal transcript expression profiles and were found to be very similar [10]. In recent years, because of the progress in understanding the immunopathogenesis of EoE, genes important for the immune responses have been target of the so called candidate gene approach. For example, a case control study identified a single nucleotide polymorphism (SNP) in a specific region of the Eotaxin-3 gene, which was found to be associated with EoE [11]. Besides the candidate gene approach, a genomewide association study revealed a locus on chromosome 5q22 that was strongly associated with EoE [12]. Polymorphisms in this locus have already been associated with other atopic diseases and peripheral eosinophilia.

Aeroallergen and Food Sensitization

Paediatric patients with EoE commonly have aeroallergen sensitization and more than 70% have elevated total IgE. Children are sensitized to both outdoor and indoor allergens with reports of 26% and 37% of patients allergic to grass and *Alternaria* respectively, and 16-19% sensitized to cockcroach and house dust mite allergens [13, 14]. Similar to adults, there can be seasonal variations in the diagnosis and severity of EoE in children [15]. Despite these observations, a definitive link between pollen and human pediatric EoE remains unclear. Further studies that document the pattern of aeroallergen sensitization with the season of EoE onset and/or exacerbation are required. In contrast to adults, the majority of children with EoE have food sensitization. Serum IgE detects more positive tests than skin prick testing, but the clinical utility and significance of this detection remains unclear. Currently, there is paucity of interventional data that use serum food-specific IgE levels as the basis for food elimination diets. In order to detect potential delayed-type food hypersensitivity reactions, atopy patch testing to food has been introduced in EoE.

The combination of food prick and patch testing has been reported to have high rates of success in predicting antigens that trigger EoE [16]. While positive patch testing may aid in the creation of a directed elimination diet, standardization and validation of patch testing in EoE is needed. Studies using prick, patch and IgE serum testing for foods have found certain foods in common that are positive by all three test procedures in children, in particular milk, egg and wheat [14]. Combined prick and patch testing additionally find corn, beef, chicken, barley, oat and rice as common positive tests. Interestingly, an empiric elimination diet (milk, egg, soy, wheat, peanuts, tree nuts, fish, shellfish) followed by reintroduction demonstrates that milk, egg, soy and wheat are the four main EoE triggers in children.

Clinical Manifestations

Clinical symptoms vary according to age. In infants and toddlers EoE mainly presents with nonspecific symptoms such as irritability, vomiting, regurgitation, feeding refusal which can result in failure to thrive [2]. During childhood vomiting, abdominal pain and more rarely retrosternal pain are reported. In paediatric age, in particular in young children dysphagia and all the feeding dysfunctions can be subtle and often difficult for the clinician to identify. These symptoms can be concealed through coping mechanisms such as the avoidance of high textured foods, cutting food in small pieces, softening food with liquids and prolonged chewing [18]. In fact, children often develop coping strategies to avoid symptoms; when asked whether swallowing is problematic they might respond ‘no’, but when further questions are posed, such as ‘Do you wash down food with liquid?’, ‘Are you the last one to leave the table?’ ‘Do you chew your food for a long time?’, the answer is often ‘yes’, indicating a compensatory behavior. Moreover, the clinical picture may be difficult to assess in children, particularly in infants and young learning-disabled children who are unable to provide accurate information on their symptoms. In adolescence symptoms become more similar to those of adulthood, represented by gastroesophageal reflux symptoms (heartburn, chest pain), dysphagia and food impaction [19]. Dysphagia is typically for solids and in cases of severe esophageal narrowing it can also be for liquids. Symptoms are more prominent and swallowing disturbances more pronounced when the ingested food's consistency is dry or rough and /or when the patients eats too fast. During the disease course, more than one third of untreated EoE patients will experience long-lasting food impactions that require endoscopic bolus removal. EoE is the main cause of food impaction in young male patients.

Natural History and Prognosis

EoE is considered a chronic and relapsing inflammatory disease which requires prolonged therapy and has a poor correlation between the clinical symptoms and the histological findings. In fact, a histological persistence of eosinophil infiltration has been observed in some patients, despite favorable clinical response. There is evidence that inhaled aeroallergens (including pollens and molds) can trigger symptom relapse, resulting in seasonal exacerbation in atopic patients, often characterized by food bolus impaction [2].

Data on the natural history of EoE are scanty. A large cohort studied conducted in children and adults by Dellon et at showed that an inflammatory phenotype was more common in the younger age and a fibro-stenotic phenotype was more frequent in adulthood [20]. This finding suggested a possible progression from an inflammatory to a fibrostenotic condition as natural history of EoE.

To date, little is known about the impact of medical intervention on the progression of disease, it has been hypothesized that early treatment may decrease the progression to fibrostenotic phenotype. Although EoE is considered a chronic and relapsing disease, its prognosis is difficult to define, as long-term data are available only in selected individuals. A long-term follow-up of >500 children treated with different regimes showed that only 11 patients maintained remission on a normal diet and off treatment. In the same study, a subgroup of 24 children, in which the family had refused any type of intervention, showed no histological improvement during a 6.2 ± 3.6 years follow-up with symptoms worsening over time, including food impaction and dysphagia [21].

Endoscopic Features

Typical endoscopic findings include esophageal rings, a thickened, often pale mucosa with linear furrows, white exudates, fixed esophageal rings (trachealization or corrugated rings) and less often narrowing of the caliber of the esophagus [22].

Mucosal breaks (erosions or ulcerations) are not typical findings of EoE and are suggestive for other conditions such as gastroesophageal reflux disease (GERD) or Crohn's disease. A normal esophagus at endoscopy does not exclude the diagnosis of EoE. To maximize diagnostic sensitivity it is recommended that at least 2 to 4 biopsies should be taken from both the proximal and distal esophagus, regardless of the endoscopic appearance of the esophagus.

The rational of obtaining biopsies from both proximal and distal esophagus is that in EoE the histological abnormalities, in particular the eosinophil infiltrate, tends to be panesophageal.

Histopathological Features

Eosinophils are not normally found in the esophageal mucosa and the quantity of intraepithelial eosinophils is a crucial component in the diagnosis of EoE. The lower threshold, for the diagnosis of EoE, is the presence of 15 eosinophils per high power field (hpf). Besides mucosal eosinophilia, histological findings include basal cell proliferation, lamina propria fibrosis and occasionally eosinophilic microabscesses. Other inflammatory cells are also found in EoE biopsies, mast cells and basophils. However, there are some controversies regarding histological diagnosis. Firstly, the lack of standardization of hpf, may alter the sensitivity and specificity of the lower threshold. Secondly, the mucosal biopsies, considered as diagnostic are often predominantly if not entirely epithelial and this may underestimate a deeper involvement in the subepithelial tissues, where eosinophil recruitment generally begins.

Furthermore, there are other histological abnormalities that occur in subepithelial layers, such as esophageal wall thickening, fibrosis and neural dysfunction, which are not identified by means of the epithelial biopsies. Table 1 summarizes both the macroscopical appearance and histological findings suggestive for EoE.

Table 1. The most common macroscopical and histological features of EoE

Macroscopical appearance	Histological findings
Normal esophagus	Eosinophil microabscesses
Stacked circular rings	Superficial layering of eosinophils
Strictures	Sheets of eosinophils
Attenuation of the subepithelial vascular pattern	Extracellular eosinophil granules
Linear furrows	Subepithelial and lamina propria fibrosis and Inflammation
Whitish papules	Basal cell hyperplasia
Small caliber esophagus	Papillary lengthening

Diagnosis

According to the current ESPGHAN guidelines, EoE can be diagnosed in presence of the following criteria [2].

- Symptoms of esophageal dysfunction (food impaction, dysphagia, vomiting, heartburn, feeding intolerance)
- Presence of 15 or more eosinophils per hpf on esophageal biopsy
- The disease interests only the esophagus and other causes of esophageal eosinophilia must be excluded

Laboratory Tests

In EoE peripheral eosinophilia (>700 cells/mm^3) and elevated immunoglobulin E (IgE) have been found, due to a sensitization to food or environmental antigens that maybe the triggers of the disease. Since the food is often reputed as the triggering element and the dietary elimination is one of the cardinal therapy, it is important to identify the right elements responsible, to avoid excessive diet; for this purpose SPT and APT are performed. These tests are reliable for the negative predictive value, but have a poor positive predictive value [2].

Allergy Testings

Skin Prick Testing

Current clinical practice for allergic evaluation of patients with EoE relies on SPT because the use of food-specific serum IgE has not been standardized. Spergel et al. have defined the diagnostic accuracy of SPT in children with EoE [23, 24]. The positive predictive values (PPVs) of SPT and APT were calculated for the 12 most common foods causing EoE [24]. The PPV for SPT was greater than 75% for milk, egg, beef and peanuts. The predictive value for APT ranged from 94% for beef to 54% for potato. Furthermore, the combination of SPT and APT showed to have an excellent negative predictive value (NPV), ranging from 88%-100% for all food types, except milk which was very low, 41%. The positive predictive value for the combined test was greater than 74% for the most common foods causing EoE (milk, egg and soy) [24]. Therefore, the combination of SPT and APT in designing a diet plan has a high success rate for food elimination and food reintroduction in EoE.

Atopy Patch Testing to Food Allergens

Atopy patch testing aims to assess cellular responses to epicutaneous exposure of food allergens. The interpretation of APT is largely subjective and prone to interobserver variation. A negative APT often does not exclude a food allergen (low sensitivity), while a strong positive test adds weight to the decision to eliminate a food from the diet. Spergel et al. has defined the diagnostic properties for the APT, although the usefulness of the APT is not universally accepted [23, 24]. To date, APT to aeroallergens (grass, pollen or house dust mite) has not been investigated yet in the context of EoE. Further studies to define the diagnostic accuracy of APT are required.

Radiology

Barium studies can be helpful for indentifying anatomic abnormalities in EoE such as strictures and ringed esophagus. Other diagnostic tests, including endoscopic ultrasound, impedance planimetry and esophageal manometry are still not considered for routinary use.

Differential Diagnosis

The main differential diagnosis of EoE is with GERD, although other diseases that are also associated with esophageal eosinophilia should also be excluded (Table 2).

The relation between EoE and GERD is complex. These two conditions share similar clinical presentation and histological findings [25]. They are not mutually exclusive and sometimes one condition predisposes and/or exacerbates the other.

On one hand, GERD with mucosal breaks (erosions and ulcerations) may impair the barrier function and increase the risk for food sensitization. This mechanism may explain the reason why patients with increased risk for GERD, for example children after esophageal atresia repair, have an increased risk for developing EoE. On the other hand, the inflammatory and eosinophil infiltrate may induce esophageal dysmotility, increasing the number of transient lower esophageal sphincter relaxations and impairing esophageal clearance, promoting GERD. The differentiation between GERD and EoE based on clinical symptoms remains a challenge in pediatrics.

The lack of response to an 8 week trial with proton pump inhibitors (PPIs) and/or the absence of significant reflux events with esophageal pH-impedance monitoring supports a diagnosis of EoE. Recently, Mulder et al. proposed a scoring system based on clinical and endoscopic features to differentiate EoE from GERD which may be useful in older children and adolescents [26]. Furthermore, a differentiation may be done by means of immunohistochemical staining for intraepithelial mast-cells and IgE-bearing cells [27].

Table 2. Conditions associated with esophageal eosinophilia

Causes of esophageal eosinophilia	
Gastroesophageal reflux disease (GERD)	Hypereosinophilic syndrome
Esophageal achalasia	Graft-versus-host-disease
Infectious esophagitis	Vasculitis
Crohn's disease	Drug sensitivity
Coeliac disease	Connective tissue disease

Proton Pump Inhibitor Responsive Esophageal Eosinophilia (PPI-REE) and Role of Antisecretory Drugs

Recently, a new clinical entity has been defined as "Proton Pump inhibitor responsive Eosinophilic esophagitis (PPI-REE)". This condition is characterized histologically by esophageal eosinophilia and clinically by symptoms of esophageal dysfunction which improve after treatment with PPIs [28, 29]. The mechanisms underlying the clinical response to PPIs esophageal eosinophilia are still unknown. It has been hypothesized that PPIs can modulate inflammatory status, inhibiting a proinflammatory response [2].

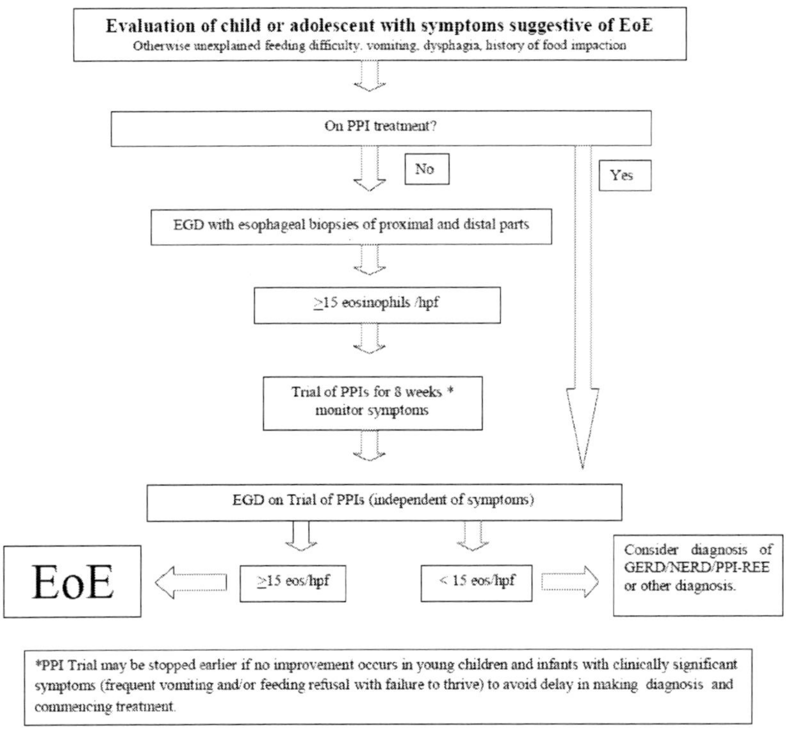

Figure 1. Algorithm for evaluation of children and adolescents with symptoms suggestive for EoE. EGD= esophagogastroduodenoscopy, eos/hpf= eosinophils per high power field, GERD= gastroesophageal reflux disease, NERD= non erosive gastroesophageal reflux disease, PPIs= proton pump inhibitors, PPI-REE= proton pump inhibitor-responsive esophageal eosinophilia. Modified from ESPGHAN Eosinophilic Esophagitis Working Group and the Gastroenterology Committee. Management guidelines of eosinophilic esophagitis in childhood, *J. Pediatr. Gastroenterol. Nutr.* 2014 Jan [2].

In children and adolescents symptomatic for esophageal dysfunction and with histological findings of esophageal eosinophilia, a trial of PPIs is recommended for 8 weeks, to identify patients with PPI-REE and to avoid unnecessary elimination diets and drugs.

The dosage of PPIs usually ranges between 1-2 mg/kg/day, with maximum dose 20 to 40 mg once or twice a day. After the trial with PPI an esophagogastroduodenoscopy (EGD) should be performed to assess endoscopic and histological improvement. If histology is still suggestive of EoE and other causes of esophageal eosinophilia are excluded the diagnosis of EoE can be confirmed. Figure 1 shows a proposed algorithm for the evaluation of children and adolescents with symptoms suggestive of EoE, modified from ESPGHAN working group guidelines.

Treatment

There are different therapeutic options for EoE, including dietary and pharmaceutical interventions. Figure 2 shows a proposed algorithm for the therapeutic management of children with EoE [1, 2]. Ideally, a successful treatment should induce both clinical and histological remission. Although there are no follow-up studies assessing the long-term consequences of esophageal eosinophilia in symptom-free patients, the possibility of a fibrostenotic process in asymptomatic patients cannot be excluded.

Elimination Diets

Many studies have shown the success of elimination diet in resolution of the symptoms and in the normalization of the biopsies, with a normal eosinophil counts and should always be considered in children as a therapeutic option, at least for 4 to 12 weeks. There are mainly three dietary approaches represented by amino acid-based formula diet, targeted elimination diet and empiric elimination diet.

- Aminoacid-based formula (AAF), for 4 weeks, was the first approach to be proposed more than 15 years ago in children diagnosed with GERD, which persisted despite treatment (medical and surgical) and improved after the AAF. Due to the severe food restriction implied, this approach is accepted more in infants than in older children and adolescents; however it's recommended in children with multiple allergies, failure to thrive and severe disease, not responding to a multiple elimination diet.

- Targeted Elimination Diet (TED) has a long term tolerability and uses the elimination of food detected by SPTs and APT. The most common foods, found out to be a trigger, are milk protein, egg, peanuts, soy, grains (wheat, rice, corn, oats) and meat (beef, chicken, turkey, pork). Currently, it is proposed for 8 -12 weeks. In some studies it has shown to be not successful, probably due to the inability of SPTs and APT to find out the real triggers. However some Authors proposed the elimination of the cow's milk protein, regardless the allergies testing, in infants and toddlers until 3 years given that it is considered one of the most common food antigen and cause of food allergies [2].
- Empiric Elimination diet (EED), for at least 8 to 12 weeks, rests on the avoidance of the 6 food accepted like the most allergenic (cow's milk, egg, wheat,soy, peanuts, fish/shellfish), without any known food sensitization.

All the three approaches are to be supervised by dietitian to maintain a correct nutritional balance and to reduce the non adherence to the diet. A critical point is the lack of a standard duration of the dietary therapy, useful to achieve the remission; AAF seems to achieve clinical and histological remission sooner than TED and EED.

If diet is successful, foods can be reintroduced at time, depending on each patient's situation, with careful follow up to avoid relapsing of the symptoms [2].

Non Dietary Interventions

Corticosteroids

Corticosteroid treatment can be extremely effective at inducing remission in patients with EoE even though treatment discontinuation often results in symptom relapse.

To date, topical corticosteroids for 4-12 weeks, alone or in combination with dietary interventions, is considered the first line treatment for induction of remission of EoE in children [2]. The two main topical corticosteroids are fluticasone proprionate (FP) and oral viscous budesonide (OBV). When swallowed, they are both safe and effective at achieving resolution of symptoms. The main adverse effect is esophageal candidiasis, which responds well to antifungal treatment.

- Fluticasone propionate (FP). A small open-label cohort study of 11 children with EoE showed that swallowed FP achieved a significant reduction in the number of eosinophils as well as CD3+ and CD8+ lymphocytes in proximal and distal esophageal mucosa [30]. In a large clinical controlled trial 36 children were randomly assigned to receive swallowed FP (880µg in 2 divided doses) or placebo for 3-months period. In these children, a resolution of symptoms occurred in 67% of subjects receiving swallowed FP and in 27% of those receiving placebo, whereas histological remission was found in 50% and 9% respectively [31]. The recommended dosage of swallowed FP is 88 to 440µg 2 to 4 times daily in children and 440 to 880µg in adolescents and adults. It is also suggested that patients swallow the dose that is delivered in the oral cavity and (and not inhaled), then not eat, drink or rinse their mouth for 30 minutes.
- Oral viscous budesonide (OVB). The first double-blind randomized controlled trial was carried out in 24 children with EoE in whom a 3-month treatment with OVB was compared to placebo. Eleven of these patients were food sensitized/allergic children. OVB was associated with improvement of symptoms in 86.7% of children, whereas no patient improved while receiving placebo. Esophageal eosinophil count decreased significantly in patients receiving OVB but not in those receiving placebo [32]. The optimal dose of OVB in children with EoE has not been formally defined. Gupta et al. evaluated the efficacy and safety of different doses of OVB in treating children with EoE in the Paediatric Eosinophilic Esophagitis Research (PEER) study [33]. The study showed a significant higher percentage of responders in children who received higher doses of OVB compared to placebo. Furthermore, there was a significant dose-related histological improvement in children receiving higher doses of OVB compared to placebo. Low-dose OVB proved to have no/minimal effect on clinical and histological parameters. Based on available evidence, the recommended starting dose of budesonide as a viscous suspension is 1 mg/daily for children <10 years of age and 2 mg/daily for older children and adults divided in 2 doses. If there is no improvement, the dose can be increased to 2,8 mg and to 4 mg respectively.

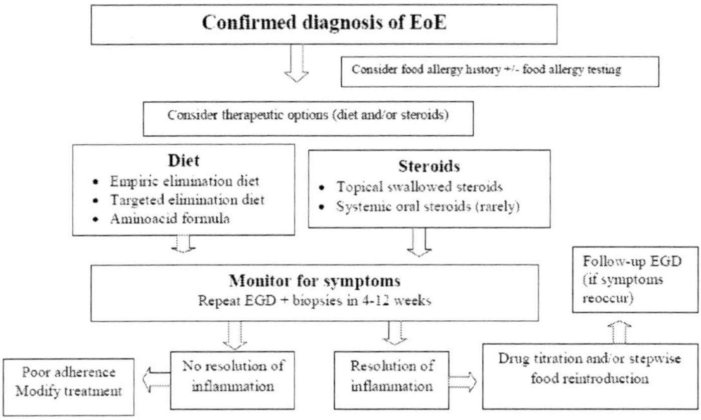

Figure 2. Algorithm for the management of children and adolescents with EoE. EGD= esophagogastroduodenoscopy. Modified from ESPGHAN Eosinophilic Esophagitis Working Group and the Gastroenterology Committee. Management guidelines of eosinophilic esophagitis in childhood, *J. Pediatr. Gastroenterol. Nutr.* 2014 Jan (2).

Systemic Corticosteroids

Oral corticosteroids are extremely effective at symptom control, but they are rarely used in patients with EoE due to the long-term side effects. However, systemic corticosteroids can be used when immediate relief of severe symptoms may be required. For example in case of severe vomiting with dehydration, dysphagia, severe food impaction with weight loss. Furthermore, oral steroids may be used when other formulations have been unsuccessful. However, the relative thickness of the esophageal epithelial barrier, compared with that of the lung, together with the recruitment pattern of eosinophils, starting from the deeper, subepithelial layers may suggest that topical treatment alone may be less effective than in asthma and that courses of oral steroids may be useful in selected cases with treatment-resistant exacerbations. Their dose is similar to that used in inflammatory bowel disease (1-2 mg/kg/daily of prednisolone orally with a maximum of 40 mg/daily). This dose should be weaned down gradually.

Other Treatment Options

Immunomodulators and Biologics

Other known medications for EoE are sodium cromoglycate, leukotriene receptor antagonist, immunomodulators and biologics (Resilizumab,

Omalizumab, anti-TNF agents). There is inadequate evidence on safety and efficacy of sodium cromoglycate and leukotriene receptor antagonist, hence, to date they are not recommended as treatment for children with EoE.

In view of the inability of corticosteroids in maintaining long-term remission, immunomodulation has been considered as a potential means of providing maintenance treatment. A trial of thiopurines in 3 patients with EoE, who were resistant to corticosteroids, proved effective in achieving symptom resolution and maintaining remission [34]. However, their use has not been further studied, hence they cannot be recommended yet. Resilizumab, a humanized monoclonal antibody with potent IL-5 neutralizing effects has been evaluated in a double-blind trial involving 226 paediatric patients, receiving 4 doses of treatment. Resilizumab was able to reduce the esophageal eosinophilia but no correlation was found between the histological and clinical improvement [35]. Omalizumab is a humanized anti-IgE antibody that binds IgE, thus preventing activation of mast cells and basophils. This antibody has been studied in adults with controversial results, no clinical trial has yet been conducted in children. A recent case report of 2 children with EoE and multiple food allergies showed that omalizumab was effective in improving food tolerance and symptoms but did not improve endoscopic or histological abnormalities [36]. Tumor necrosis factor (TNF) has been found to be more highly expressed in epithelial cells of active EoE compared to normal esophageal mucosa [37]. This observation lead to hypothesize that anti-TNF agents could have a useful role in treatment of EoE. However, a recent report on 3 adult with severe, cortico-steroid-dependent EoE treated with 2 doses of Infliximab showed only mild improvement of symptoms [38].

Esophageal Dilatation

Esophageal dilatation can be useful in children who present with severe esophageal stricture, in case there has been no response to medical treatment. Most of the data on esophageal dilatation regards EoE in adults [39]. In a recent review of 13 pediatric patients, dilatations were performed in 4 cases with good results [40]. The specific techniques, balloon or boogie dilatation, seem to be equally effective with a risk of perforation equal to 1%.

Future Directions and Future Research

Further studies are required to show whether the diagnosis of EoE can be assumed without PPI treatment in older children and adolescents with typical symptoms of dysphagia or food impaction and typical endoscopic and histological findings of EoE. Well-designed prospective randomized studies of PPIs vs placebo are required in treatment-naïve children with esophageal eosinophilia, without additional dietary intervention.

There are few high quality randomized studies assessing the efficacy of different pharmaceutical agents, other than corticosteroids, in paediatric EoE. Prospective intervention studies would be very useful to achieve a more uniform, evidence-based approach to non dietary interventions in EoE treatment. Future potential therapeutic options for EoE include anti-IL-5 receptor monocolonal antibodies, which have been shown to decrease peripheral eosinophilia in patients with asthma [41]. Furthermore, local treatment targeted at inhibition of IL-4 and IL-13 is under study for treatment of asthma and could be useful also in the field of EoE. A better understanding of disease phenotype, natural history and the mechanisms underlying treatment response should lead to more effective short and long-term interventions.

Key Points

- Eosinophilic Esophagitis (EoE) is an immune/antigen-mediated esophageal disease.
- The clinical course is chronic and relapsing.
- Histologically EoE is characterized by eosinophil-predominat inflammation and clinically by symptoms of esophageal dysfunction.
- Symptoms vary according to age. In infants symptoms may be nonspecific such as irritability and food refusal. In children vomiting and abdominal pain are common. In adolescents typical symptoms are dysphagia and food impaction.
- Typical endoscopic findings are represented by linear furrows, white plaques and esophageal narrowing.
- The main histological feature is eosinophil infiltrate: $\geq$ 15 eosinophils /hpf
- In symptomatic children with histological findings of esophageal eosinophilia, a trial of PPIs is recommended for 8 weeks.
- A second EGD is recommended under PPI therapy, in all children, even if the symptoms resolve.
- Dietary intervention and/or topical corticosteroids are the first line treatment of EoE.

References

[1] Liacouras CA, Furuta GT, Hirano I, et al. Eosinophilic esophagitis: updated consensus recommendations for children and adults, *J. Allergy Clin. Immunol.* 2011; 128: 3-20.

[2] Papadopoulou A, Koletzko S, Heuschkel R, et al. ESPGHAN Eosinophilic Esophagitis Working Group and the Gastroenterology Committee. Management guidelines of eosinophilic esophagitis in childhood, *J. Pediatr. Gastroenterol. Nutr.* 2014; 58: 107-18.

[3] Dellon ES, Jensen ET, Martin CF, Shaheen NJ, Kappelman MD. Prevalence of Eosinophilic Esophagitis in the United States. *Clin. Gastroenterol. Hepatol.* 2013; S1542-3565(13)01304-9.

[4] Noel RJ, Putnam PE, Rothenberg ME. Eosinophilic esophagitis. *N. Eng. J. Med.* 2004; 351: 940-1.

[5] van Rhijn BD, Smout AJ, Bredenoord AJ. Rapidly increasing incidence of eosinophilic esophagitis in a large cohort. *Neurogastroenterol. Motil.* 2013; 25: 47-52.

[6] Dellon ES. Eosinophilic esophagitis: diagnostic tests and criteria. *Curr. Opin. Gastroenterol.* 2012; 28: 382-8.

[7] Moawad FJ, Veerapan GR, Lake JM, et al. Correlation between eosinophilic esophaagitis and aeroallergens. *Aliment Pharmacol. Ther.* 2010; 31: 509-15.

[8] Franciosi JP, Tam V, Liacouras CA, Spergel JM. A case-control study of sociodemographic and geographic characteristics of 335 children with eosinophilic esophagitis. *Clin. Gastroenterol. Hepatol.* 2009; 7: 415-419.

[9] Putnam PE. Gastrointest endoscopy. *Clin. N. Am.* 2008; 18: 11-23.

[10] Collins MH, Blanchard C, Abonia JP, et al. Clinical, pathologic and molecular characterization of familial eosinophilic esophagitis compared with sporadic cases. *Clin. Gastroenterol. Hepatol.* 2008; 6:621-629.

[11] Blanchard C, Wang N, Stringer KF, et al. Eotaxin-3 and a uniquely conserved gene expression profile in eosinophilic esophagitis. *J. Clin. Invest.* 2006; 116: 536-547.

[12] Rothenberg ME, Spergel JM, Sherrill JD, et al. Common variants at 5q22 asociate with pediatric eosinophilic esophagitis. *Nat. Genet.* 2010; 42: 289-291.

[13] Onbasi K, Sin AZ, Doganavsargil B, Onder GF, Bor S, Sebik F. Eosinophil infiltration of the esophageal mucosa in patients with pollen allergy during the season. *Clin. Exp. Allergy.* 2005; 35: 1423-1431.

[14] Rayapudi M, Mavi P, Zhu X, Pandey AK, Abonia JP, Rothenberg ME et al. Indoor insect allergens are potent inducers of experimental eosinophilc esophagitis in mice. *J. Leukoc. Biol.* 2010; 88: 337-346.

[15] Wang FY, Gupta SK, Fitzgerald JF. Is there a seasonal variation in the incidence or intensity of allergic eosinophilic esophagitis in newly diagnosed children? *J. Clin. Gastroenterol.* 2007; 41: 451-453.

[16] Spergel JM, Brown-Whitehorn TF, Beausoleil Jl, et al. 14 years of eosinophilc esophagitis: clinical features and prognosis. *J. Paediatr. Gastroenterol. and Nutr.* 2009; 48: 30-36.

[17] Erwin EA, James HR, Gutekunst HM, Russo JM, Kelleher KJ, Platts-Mills TA. Serum IgE measurement and detection of food allergy in pediatric patients with eosinopilic esophagitis. *Ann. Allergy Asthma Immunol.* 2010; 104: 496-502.

[18] Dellon ES. Eosinophilic esophagitis. *Gastroenterol. Clin. North Am.* 2013;42:133-53.

[19] Dellon ES, Gonsalves N, Hirano I, Furuta GT, Liacouras CA, Katzka DA; American College of Gastroenterology, ACG clinical guideline: Evidenced based approach to the diagnosis and management of esophageal eosinophilia and eosinophilic esophagitis (EoE). *Am. J. Gastroenterol.* 2013. 108; 5: 679-92.

[20] Dellon ES, Kim HP, Sperry SL, Rybnicek DA, Woosley JT, Shaheen NJ. A phenotypic analysis shows that eosinophilic esophagitis is a progressive fibrostenotic disease. *Gastrointest. Endosc.* 2013. S0016-5107(13)02460-7.

[21] Prasad GA, Alexander JA, Schleck CD, et al. Epidemiology of eosinophilc esophagitis over three decades in Olmsted County, Minnesota. *Clin. Gastroenterol. Hepatol.* 2009; 7: 1055-1061.

[22] Dellon ES. Diagnosis and management of eosinophilic esophagitis, *Clin. Gastroenterol. Hepatol.* 2012; 10: 1066-78.

[23] Spergel JM, Beausoleil JL, Mascarenhas M, et al. The use of skin prick tests and patch tests to identify causative foods in eosinophilic esophagitis. *J. Allergy Clin. Immunol.* 2002; 109: 363-8.

[24] Spergel JM, Brown- Whitehorn T, Beausoleil Jl, et al. Predictive values for skin prick test and atopy patch test for eosinophilic esophagitis. *J. Allergy Clin. Immunol.* 2007; 119: 509-11.

[25] Fell JM, Recognition, assessment and management of eosinophilic oesophagitis. *Arch. Dis. Child.* 2013; 9:702-6.

[26] Mulder DJ, Hurlbut DJ, Noble AJ, et al. Clinical features distinguish eosinophilic ad reflux-induced esophagitis: an age-matched case-

controlled study and a novel scoring system. *J. Paediatr. Gastroenterol. Nutr.* 2013; 56: 263- 70.

[27] Kirsch R, Bokhary R, Marcon MA, et al. Activated mucosal mast cells differentiate eosinophilic (allergic) esophagitis from gastroesophageal reflux disease. *J. Paediatr. Gastroenterol. Nutr.* 2013; 56: 263-70.

[28] Dellon ES, Speck O, Woodward K, et al. Clinical and Endoscopic Characteristics do Not Reliably Differentiate PPI-Responsive Esophageal Eosinophilia and Eosinophilic Esophagitis in Patients Undergoing Upper Endoscopy: A Prospective Cohort Study, *Am. J. Gastroenterol.* 2013. 108; 12:1854-60.

[29] Moawad FJ, Schoepfer AM, Safroneeva E, et al. Eosinophilic oesophagitis and proton pump inhibitor-responsive oesophageal eosinophilia have similar clinical, endoscopic and histological findings. *Aliment. Pharmacol. Ther.* 2014; Jan 26. doi: 10.1111/apt.12636.

[30] Teitelbaum JE, Fox VL, Twarog FJ, et al. Eosinophilc esophagitis in children: immunopathological analysis and response to fluticasone proprionate. *Gastroenterology* 2002; 122: 1216-25.

[31] Konikoff MR, Noel RJ, Blanchard C et al. A randomized, double-blind, placebo-controlled trial of fluticasone proprionate for pediatric eosinophilic esophagitis. *Gastroenterology* 2006; 131: 1381-1391.

[32] Dohil R, Newbury RO, Fox L, et al. Oral viscous budesonide is effective in children with eosinophilic esophagitis in a randomized placebo-controlled trial. *Gastroenterology* 2010; 139: 418-429.

[33] Gupta SK, Collins MH, Lewis JD, et al. Efficacy and safety of oral budesonide suspension (OBS) in pediatric subjects with eosinophilic esophagitis (EoE): results from the double-blind placebo- controlled PEER study. *Gastroenterology* 2011; 140: S179.

[34] Netzer P, Gschossmann JM, Straumann A, et al. Corticosteroid dependent eosinophilic esophagitis: azathioprine and 6-mercaptopurine can induce and maintain long-term remission. *Eur. J. Gastroenterol. Hepatol.* 2007; 19:865–9.

[35] Spergel JM, Rothenberg ME, Collins MH, et al. Reslizumab in children and adolescents with eosinophilic esophagitis:results of a double-blind, randomised placebo controlled trial. *J. Allergy Clin. Immunol.* 2012; 129:456–63.

[36] Rocha R, Vitor AB, Trindade E, et al. Omalizumab in the treatment of eosinophilic esophagitis and food allergy. *Eur. J. Pediatr.* 2011; 170: 1471– 4.

[37] Straumann A, Bauer M, Fischer B, et al. Idiopathic eosinophilic esophagitis is associated with a T(H)2-type allergic inflammatory response. *J. Allergy Clin. Immunol.* 2001; 108:954–61.

[38] Straumann A, Bussmann C, Conus S, et al. Anti-TNF-alpha (infliximab) therapy for severe adult eosinophilic esophagitis. *J. Allergy Clin. Immunol.* 2008; 122:425–7.

[39] Schoepfer AM, Gschossmann J, Scheurer U, et al. Esophageal strictures in adult eosinophilic esophagitis: dilation is an effective and safe alternative after failure of topical corticosteroids. *Endoscopy* 2008; 40:161–4.

[40] Robles-Medranda C, Villard F, le Gall C, et al. Severe dysphagia in children with eosinophilic esophagitis and esophageal stricture: an indication for balloon dilation? *J. Pediatr. Gastroenterol. Nutr.* 2010; 50:516–20.

[41] Wenzel S, Wilbraham D, Fuller R, et al. Effect of an interleukin-4 variant on late phase asthmatic response to allergen challenge in asthmatic patients: results of two phase 2a studies. *Lancet* 2007; 370:1422–31.

In: Eosinophilia
Editor: Rosanna Finlay
ISBN: 978-1-63321-355-5

Chapter 3

Approach to a Child with Eosinophilia

Chiara Mameli, Silvia Mauri, Valentina Giudici, Matteo Torcoletti and Gian Vincenzo Zuccotti
Department of Pediatrics, L. Sacco Hospital, University of Milan, Italy

Abstract

Eosinophilis are important cells in inflammatory processes, organ and tissue injury and fibrosis. Eosinophilia, resulting from increased bone marrow poiesis and subsequent tissue accumulation, can cause a broad and variegate spectrum of disorders (infectious, connective, allergic, neoplastic and idiopathic disease). In developed countries allergic or atopic disorders are prevailing among paediatric population. A classification of hypereosinophilia based on eosinophilis count has been established: mild form (351-1500/mmc), moderate form (1501-5000/mmc) and severe form (>5000/mmc). An increase in tissue eosinophilia may be seen with or without concomitant peripheral eosinophilia. Clinical presentation and degree of eosinophilia may be very different in relation to the organ which is involved. An higher risk of complications has been described in moderate to severe forms independently from aetiology and is related to tissue and organ infiltration. A detailed medical and familiar history including gastrointestinal, atopic, infective and systemic symptoms should be recorded, including possible recent travel and use of medications.

Physical examination should include cardiorespiratory and abdominal evaluation with attention to masses and haepatosplenomegaly and search for dysmorphisms, lymphonodal and articolar involvement and dermatologic lesions (eg: rash, signs of haemorragic diathesis). In the clinical approach to a child with eosinophilia first level blood examination (blood cell counts, coagulation profile, haepatic and renal function, inflammatory markers and immunoglobulin) can help in discriminating the possible aetiology and therefore guide the second level examinations (specific allergic tests, immunologic, infectious and onco-haematological work-up). When an underlying cause is not identified idiopathic hypereosinophilia must be considered and at present, a diagnosis of primary eosinophilia mandates a bone marrow examination, karyotype analysis, and molecular studies. The treatment of secondary eosinophilia depends on the aetiology and therefore demands the therapeutic option to a specific setting. In case of idiopathic hypereosinophilia instead, the therapy includes steroids as first line, hydroxyurea, interferon-alpha, chemoterapeuthics and monoclonal antibodies as second line. Allogeneic transplantation offers a viable treatment option for drug-refractory cases.

Introduction

Eosinophilia is a common finding in clinical practice and can serve as a useful clue for differential diagnosis when found in association with a constellation of signs and symptoms. Disorders involved in eosinophilia range from mild, self-limited to severe, life-threatening diseases. Worldwide, parasitic infections are the most common cause of eosinophilia; however, allergic disease is the prevailing cause in industrialized countries. Additional causes of more pronounced eosinophilia include variant hypereosinophilic syndromes (HES) that merit consideration based on recent newer diagnostic and therapeutic options. The presenting symptomatology and spectrum of eosinophilic diseases in children can differ from those seen in adults; in this chapter we outline the major causes, clinical presentation, diagnostic approach and principle of treatment of eosinophilia in pediatric population.

Eosinophils Cells Biology

Eosinophils are multifunctional leukocytes which have their predominant function in innate immunity, inflammation processes and more in general in host responses. They differentiate in the bone marrow and this process is regulated by specific transcription factors. Eosinophils maturation occurs in response to eosinophilopoietic cytokines, such as interleukin 3 (IL-3), granulocyte-macrophage colony stimulating factor (GM-CSF) and interleukin 5 (IL-5) [1]. In particular IL-5 shares with eosinophils a common β chain in their receptors and has been identified as the most eosinophil-specific cytokine: it is in fact IL-5 which directs the development of precursors into the eosinophil lineage, stimulates their release from bone marrow and guides eosinophils accumulation into specific tissues. In healthy subjects, eosinophils are predominantly located in the spleen, lymphnodes and gastrointestinal apparatus, with the exception of esophagus, thymus and mammary glands [2]. When in peripheral blood, eosinophils rolling along the endothelium process is mediated by interactions of P-selectin glycoprotein ligand 1 (PSGL-1) and their long term survival in peripheral tissues is mediated again by IL-3, IL-5 and GM-CSF; in the resident specific tissues eosinophils act their proinflammatiry effects via the discharge of toxic mediators and this results in direct tissue destruction via ribonuclease activity and toxic pore formation, and they also can activate the degranulation of mast cells and basophils [3].

Definition of Eosinophilia

Usually, the peripheral blood eosinophils are 1 to 3% of the total leukocytes, with an absolute count of about 350 per μL.

Eosinophilia is defined as absolute blood count exceeding $0.5 \times 10^9/l$, while hypereosinophilia refers to absolute blood count greater than $1.5 \times 10^9/l$. A classification of hypereosinophilia based on blood eosinophil count has been established, therefore eosinophilia is regarded as:

- mild (351-1500 eosinophils/μl),
- moderate (1501-5000 eosinophils/ μl)
- severe (>5000 eosinophils/μl)

Variations in the eosinophils number are seen in different disorders, as for example allergic respiratory diseases and eczema are associated with mild eosinophilia, whereas parasitic and neoplastic diseases are typically associated with more severe eosinophilia. (Table 1)

An increase in tissue eosinophilia may be seen with or without concomitant peripheral eosinophilia [3]. Whereas a modest number of eosinophils are found in normal specific tissues, their excessive infiltration may cause organ damage due to inflammation, tissue fibrosis and eosinophils release of their granule contents.

Another classification of eosinophilia can be in primary or secondary eosinophilia. A secondary or reactive increase in blood eosinophils, tissue eosinophils, or both is associated with a wide variety of infections (especially helminthic parasites), allergic responses, neoplasms, connective tissue disorders, medications and endocrinopathies.

Table 1. Eosinophilic disorders in children by degree of eosinophilia

DEGREE OF EOSINOPHILIA	EOSINOPHILIC DISORDERS
Mild (351-1500/μL cells)	Allergic rhinitis Eczema Asthma Parasitic infection Reaction to drugs Oncological disorders Occupational lung disease Gastrointestinal disease including EGID (eosinophil gastrointestinal disorder) Certain infectious diseases Long-term dialysis Radiation therapy Transplant rejection Immundeficiency state
Moderate (1501-5000/μL cells)	Parasitic infection Asthma Pulmonary eosinophilia syndrome Connective tissue disorders Reaction to drugs Oncological disorders Hypereosinophilic syndrome
Severe (> 5000/μL cells)	Parasitic infections Hypereosinophilic syndrome Eosinophilic leukemia

Adapted from: Wagelie-Steffen A, Aceves S. *Eosinophilic disorders in children. Ped Allerg Imm.* 2006; 6:475-482.

Primary eosinophilia is not a reactive phenomenon and can be described as either clonal or idiopathic in nature. If an underlying molecular or cytogenetic abnormality can be identified, the eosinophilia can be designated as a clonal disorder. If reactive causes are ruled out and no underlying clonal origin is proven, the eosinophilia is described as idiopathic [4]. In particular when a certain condition causing eosinophilia cannot be found, the Hidiopathic Hypereosinophilc Syndromes (HES) must be considered. In the past HES was previously defined as a condition characterized by (1) blood eosinophilia of 1.5 x 10^9/l or greater, lasting for more than 6 months, (2) no evidence of an underlying condition known to cause eosinophilia and (3) existence of eosinophil-mediated organ damage or dysfunction [5]. These criteria have been now revised [6,7] and currently HES definition has been redefined and criteria have been enlarged: first of all, HES is no longer defined by a 6 month duration but can be even shorter, provided other causes of eosinophilia have been excluded; the term hypereosinophilia should be used when the eosinophils count is greater than 1.5x 10^9/l on two occasions with a minimum of a 1-month interval. The exception is when the eosinophils count is greater than 1.5x 10^9/l and there is life-threatening organ dysfunction and/or tissue eosinophilia is documented. For the diagnosis, the following criteria should be met:

- eosinophils should constitute more than 20% of all nucleated cells in the bone marrow section;
- massive tissue infiltration by eosinophils should be found in tissue biopsies by pathologic study;
- specific staining should reveal local deposition of eosinophil-derived contents.

Principles Causes of Eosinophilia

Allergic and Respiratory Diseases

All children presenting with rinithis, conjunctivitis or dermatologic lesions such as eczema or dermatitis should be evaluated for the possible presence of elevated eosinophils count in peripheral blood. No particular action must be taken, except for aiming at eliminating the principle allergic cause. Among rinithis, one of the most common type which can be associated with non peripheral eosinophilia, is the Non Allergic Rinithis with Eosinophilia Syndrome (NARES). NARES is characterized by nasal and upper airways symptoms that occur without regular intervals related to specific seasons in children with negative allergic skin and blood test [8]. When a clinical suspicion of NARES is raised, nasal cytology should be provided to help the diagnosis. Of note, a subgroup of NARES syndrome, presenting with elevated peripheral eosinophils count is reported in literature; it is the so called Blood Eosinophilia Nonallergic Rinithis Syndrome (BENARS), which once again can be found in presence of negative allergen skin test and normal IgE count levels [8].

Among respiratory diseases, eosinophilic lung diseases can be found in association with peripheral or tissue eosinophilia; among these, particular attention should be given to asthma which is the most common respiratory disease in children. It is important also to mention allergic bronchopulmonary aspergillosis, a condition often associated with cystic fibrosis, even if rarely in children, acute and chronic eosinophilic pneumonia and simple pulmonary eosinophilia in context of parasitic infections or drug reactions (the most common drugs involved in these cases are ethambutol, non steroidal anti-inflammatory agents, some antibiotics such as cotrimoxazole) [9,10]. Special mention for some form of vasculitis which can involve the respiratory tract, as sometimes occur in the Churg-Strauss setting [11].

Neoplastic Diseases

Clonal causes of eosinophilia account for < 1% and include acute and chronic myeloid/lymphoid leukemia, acute and chronic eosinophilic leukemia and myeloproliferatives syndromes. Instead, the so called paraneoplastic eosinophilia can be found in association with some neoplastic disease, including adenocarcinomas of the bowel, lung, ovary or other solid organs, some forms of Hodgkin disease, T-cell lymphoma and mastocytosis [12].

Immunologic Disorders

Other infrequent causes associated with eosinophilia can be searched in the setting of primary or secondary immunodeficiency and, among them, we would like to mention rare immunodeficiency disorders, such as Iper IgE syndrome and Omenn syndrome.

Omenn's syndrome, also known as combined immunodeficiency with hypereosinophilia syndrome, is a primary recessive inherited immunodeficiency caused by a mutation of RAG1/2 genes. It is characterized by increased susceptibility to opportunistic infections, hypereosinophilia, protracted diarrhea, rashes, enlargement of the lymph nodes and the spleen. If not treated properly, Omenn's syndrome will prove fatal within the first two to six months of life [13].

Iper IgE recurrent infection syndrome is a complex immunodeficiency with multiorgan clinical manifestation. Different genetical backrground are responsible for this syndrome: classic form is inherited as autosomal dominant form and it is caused by a mutation in a transcription factor gene STAT3 (signal transducer and activator of transcription 3); this mutation leads to impairment of signaling of many cytokines, as well as dysfunction of T-Helper lymphocites which play a crucial role in immune response to infections, in particular those sustained by extracellular bacteria and fungi. From the clinical point of view, this syndrome is characterized by a classical triad of symptoms which are: recurrent abscesses of staphylococcal aetiology, recurrent respiratory tract infections and elevated serum Immunoglobulin E concentrations. Spectrum of signs and symptoms is variable and ranging from a severe form of dermatitis to skeletal, dental and connective tissue disorders [14]. A particular attention must be given to patient whom could be facing rejection in solid organ transplant and thus presenting with a Graft Versus Host Disease.

Infectious Diseases

Infectious diseases represents another common cause of hypereosinophilia that must be investigated and, among them, parasitic infections are the most common. A detailed history of the patient's habitat and geographic exposure during travels, immigration and dietary habits will help in dictate the type of parasites and to look for using serologic tests and examinations of stools, urine and blood. Among parasitic disorders we can mention infection with *Toxocara canis* that can be contracted after contact with soil or ingestion of vegetables which have been contaminated by excrement from infected dogs. Of greatest concern could be the infection with *Strongyloides stercoralis*, the infective larvae which penetrate the skin through contact with soil or water contaminated with human feces. This helmint is the only one which can propagate internally for decades after the initial infectios and therefore cause variable eosinophilia, with or without other symptoms. *S. stercoralis* is endemic in tropical and subtropical regions, especially in rural and poor socioeconomic habitats. Stool examinations for ova and parasites are mandatory in patients, even if the sensitivity for *S. stercoralis* is very low, therefore when the clinical suspect is high, patients should be screened for serum antibodies using ELISAs. Other infectious diseases which could cause elevated levels of eosinophilia are chronic tubercolosis, coccidiomycosis, scabies, aspergillosis, Malaria-fever and toxoplasmosis. Moreover infections by HIV, Ebstein Barr Virus, amoeba and *Pneumocystis carinii* can cause reactive eosinophilia [2]. In infectious diseases eosinophilia levels can fluctuate over time and any level of severity can be observed.

Gastrointestinal Disease

Gastrointestinal disorders associated with eosinophilia can be found at any different levels of the gastrointestinal tract: eosinophilic esophagitis, eosinophilic gastritis, eosinophilic gastroenteritis, eosinophilic enteritis and ulcerative colitis. The hallmark of a primary eosinophilic gastrointestinal disorders is an eosinophilic rich inflammation at any level of the gastrointestinal tract occurring in the absence of any other causes of eosinophilia [15]. To be noted that all the gastrointestinal involvement which occur distally to the esophagus tract can present without peripheral blood eosinophilia. Patients with these kind of disease can have variegate clinical presentation and diagnosis can be challenging since symptoms are quite often non specific such as failure to thrive, vomiting, diarrhea with or without protein-losing enteropathy, abdominal pain, irritability and, in particular in the setting of eosinophilic esophagitis, dysphagia [15].

Other Diseases

Eosinophilia can sometimes be found also in one of these clinical condition: hypoadrenalism, radiation exposure, systemic mastocytosis, connective tissue disorders. In particular, among other different causes of secondary eosinophilia, great attention has to be given to adverse reaction to medications, both herbal and prescribed [2]. Eosinophilia associated with adverse drug reactions is a IL-5 mediated process, and this manifestations can be subtle as sometimes can develop without any other clinical manifestations.

It has to be noted that drug-induced eosinophilia can develop without any other manifestations of adverse drug reactions, such as rashes or fevers, but should nevertheless prompt an evaluation of whether organs, including the lungs, kidneys and heart, are involved, in order to avoid harmful complications. Acute necrotizing myocarditis is an uncommon but serious type of hypersensitivity, with reactions to some medications in some cases. It can be very challenging to identify the culprit agent, especially if the patient take many medications: in clinical practice pediatricians can guided by the type of medication, as some of they are more likely responsible for an eosinophilic drug reaction than others, such as anticonvulsivants, penicillins and allopurinol.

Diagnosis can be guided also a specific target organ involvement, as for example hepatitis, skin rash, and systemic symptoms (DRESS syndrome) are more often associated with anticonvulsivants, pneumonitis with nitrofurantoin, nefritis with cephalosporin and hypersensitivity vasculitis with phentoyn [2]. In patients with drug induced pulmonary eosinophilia blood eosinophilia is usually present; when absent, bronchoalveolar lavage could be necessary to make the diagnosis clear and in patients with drug induced acute interstitial nephritis, eosinophilia is common in urine and blood.

Hypereosinophilic Syndrome Variants

Hypereosinophilic syndrome in children is a rare disease, that can occur at any age, nevertheless the incidence is unknown. Paediatric HES has a slight male predominance (55.3% male vs 44.7% female), compared with adult HES where the male:female ratio is 9:1 [16]. The presentation of the disease is variable. Different complaints like fatigue, cough, rhinitis, dispnea, itching skin rash, or even life threatening cardiac or neurologic events are observed [17].

In the paediatric population HES is commonly characterized by fever (58.8% of cases), arthralgias (23.5%), skin rash (23.5%) instead of headache and sore throat that are not very common (11.8% of cases each). These findings are quite different from the adulthood presentation, where the most common signs and symptoms are related to the respiratory tract, such as cough and dyspnea, while the less common presentation is characterized by skin rash and fever.

Tissue multiple organ damage is predominantly related to infiltration by eosinophils and release of cytokines and humoral factors; in particular organ infiltration is seen in skin, heart, lung and central nervous system. As with the adults, also in children, involvement of the cardiovascular system is the major cause of morbidity and mortality [18]. In the pediatric setting HES is quite often associated with chromosomal abnormalities, which include trisomy 8 and a *abl oncogene* translocation. In 40% of reported cases in literature so far, hypereosinophilic syndrome is associated with acute leukemia, especially acute lymphoblastic leukemia [19, 20].

The International Hypereosinophilic Syndrome Working Group recently revised the classification system for eosinophilic disorders and updated the definition according to the most recent insights of the disease; six variants have been identified and described [6]:

1) *Myeloproliferative variants* which can be also identified on the basis of clinical and laboratory findings and are characterized by pathologic evidence of eosinophil-related tissue damage and fibrosis, elevated serum triptase levels and myeloproliferative features, including haepato-splenomegaly, anemia, thrombocytopenia and increased numbers of atypical mast cells, bone marrow dysplasia, increased serum levels of cobalamin [21]. This variants include:
   a) Platelet-Derived-Growth-Factor-Receptor-α-Chain (FIP1L1-PDGFRA) associated HES
   b) unknown aetiology (FIP1L1-PDGFRA negative)
   c) chronic eosinophilic leukaemia, which is characterized by cytogenetic anomalies and/or blast on peripheral smear
2) *Lymphocitic variant* is associated with a clonal proliferation of T cells and predominantly associated with skin disease. In general this variant presents with a more benign prognosis
3) *Idiopathic/undefined variant* is not associated with chromosomal or clonal abnormalities
4) *Overlap variants* with a clinical presentation characterized by restricted organ eosinophilic disorders
5) *Associated variants* (eosinophilia associated with a defined syndrome, for example Churg-Strauss syndrome)
6) *Familial variant*: familiar history of permanent and documented hypereosinophilia of unknown aetiology.

Unfortunately, data on long term prognosis have not been reported in literature so far; it is important to know that a very early diagnosis and an intensive follow up can help the survival over the years [18].

Clinical Presentation

The combination of eosinophilia and symptoms caused by eosinophils is very important to make the correct diagnosis and give the appropriate therapy. It is generally accepted that there is no strict correlation between the degree of eosinophilia and the risk of organ-involvement and that various factors may be necessary to determine the organ damage [22].

Table 2. Organ-specific symptoms which may be caused by Eosinophilia

Organ/System	Symptoms
Heart	• Myocardial necrosis • Valvular involvement • Thrombosis and fibrosis (Loeffler's endocarditis and myocardial fibrosis in late stages) manifesting in congestive cardiac insufficiency, hypertrophy, dilation, arhythmias and effusions
Skin	• Pruritus • Urticaria • Angioedema • Mucocutaneous ulcera • Papulous or nodulous lesions
Nervous system	• Cerebral thrombosis (mostly arterial, transient ischemia, embolic or local thrombus formation) • Encephalopathy, mostly cognitive and / or upper neuron paresis. • Peripheral neuropathies.
Gastrointestinal	• Diarrhoea • Aspecific abdominal depending on a more selective localization
Pulmonary	• Chronic, generally non-productive, cough. • Bronchial hyperactivity • Pulmonary symptoms secondary to heart affection
Rheumatological	• Arthralgia (prevailing in major joints) • Arthritis • Myalgia • Raynaud's phenomenon.

Adapted from: Nordic MPD Study Group. Guidelines for the diagnosis and treatment of eosinophilia. 2nd version. 2012.

Clinical manifestations of eosinophilia are different between patients. In patients with secondary eosinophilia, the primary disease or cause may contribute to the clinical presentation. In case of primary, clonal disorders, some patients may be asymptomatic and the clinical presentation otherwise very heterogeneous [23]. Most organ-specific symptoms may be caused by the eosinophilia, and more than one organ may be involved, including the bone marrow affection in primary eosinophilia. Some organs, however, are more frequently affected in hypereosinophilic conditions (Table 2). Any symptom may be experienced in eosinophilia, for example we can see eye (for instance microthrombus formation, retinal arteritis) or renal (for instance acute renal insufficiency, glomerulopathy and glomerulonephritis) manifestations. The tissues most frequently affected by eosinophil infiltration are the heart and the skin, the nervous system and the respiratory and gastrointestinal tract in that order. The hematopoietic system is involved in every case, due to eosinophilia *per se* but neutrophilia, basophilia, dysplastic features and immature white blood cells, anemia, thrombocytopenia or thrombocytosis may also be found in blood samples and depending on the cause of eosinophilia. However, clinical symptoms cannot be related to any specific diagnose or clonal eosinophilia, since they generally represent patient populations characterized by an increased eosinophil count, but not by the same, specific diagnosis.

Clinical Examination, Laboratory Investigation and Imaging Studies

When approaching a child with eosinophilia, a clinician should first evaluate the onset, the degree of eosinophilia, the location of eosinophils accumulations (tissue, blood or both), and the clinical presentation. As already stated, a broad and variegate spectrum of disorders can be associated to eosinophilia (infectious, connective, allergic or neoplastic diseases). When dealing with a patient with eosinophilia, an accurate history should always be collected, in order to rule out possible symptoms of atopic or gastrointestinal diseases, recent travel, especially in helminth-endemic areas, drug ingestion or even general systemic symptoms (fever, weight loss, fatigue), suggestive of possible neoplastic disease.

The initial consideration of causes of eosinophilia needs to focus on several and not uncommon causes: as previously mentioned the allergic spectrum of diseases needs to be considered in children, although eosinophils count greater than $1.5 \times 10^9/l$ is uncommon in most subjects with allergy. A general physical examination should be made paying particular attention to dysmorphisms, atopic and allergic contact eczemas, rash and signs of haemorragic diathesis. When evaluating the cardiorespiratory system specific attention should be prompted to presence of cardiac murmur, wheezing, cough or breathlessness and pleuric friction rub, in the setting of possible respiratory diseases such asthma or pneumonia. Abdominal inspection focused on masses and haepatosplenomegaly is important as well as recollection of possible gastrointestinal symptoms such as abdominal pain and diarrhea, especially if the child had recent been in a helminth-endemic area. Weight loss, fever, night sweats, articular involvement and lymph nodes enlargement should be recollected, in order to underline other possible causes such as neoplastic or immune disorders [24].

Specific investigation will vary from patient to patient but the following can be recommended in all cases as first level blood examination can help in discriminating the possible aetiology and therefore guide the second level examination (Table 3). Among first level exams we include: blood cell counts, coagulation profile, haepatic and renal function, inflammatory markers and immunoglobulin. Peripheral blood smear can be useful when looking for dysplastic eosinophils or blast.

Decision on second level exams should be guided by clinical suspicion and these exams should include testing to identify viral agents, bacterial cultures and parasites search on blood and stools, specific allergic tests, immunologic and neoplastic work-up, measurement of antineutrophil cytoplasmic antibodies, serum tryptase, serum Vitamin B12, and cardiac troponin. For what concern the use of instrumental investigation, detailed non invasive evaluation of cardiothoracic (electrocardiography and echocardiography), abdominal (thoracoabdominal computed tomography scans), and cerebral district could be helpful. In some selected case tissue biopsy should be performed. When an underlying cause is not identified, despite accurate diagnostic evaluation, idiopathic hypereosinophilia must be considered and at present, a diagnosis of primary eosinophilia mandates a bone marrow examination, karyotype analysis, and additional molecular studies.

When dealing with an idiopathic eosinophilia, a bone marrow examination becomes mandatory, as well as karyotype analyses and in addition molecular studies. All these evaluation can be useful for better characterize the clinical spectrum and may help in assessing an underlying condition which could involve a possible organ damage, irrespective of the possible underlying cause the potential complications are identical.

Table 3. Testing guidelines

Investigation	Rationale
• Full blood count • Blood cell morphology	To identify the severity of eosinophilia and abnormalities in other blood cells
• IgE • Prick test • allergen specific IgE-tests	To diagnose allergic condition
• Stool parasites • Serological tests for schistosomiasis, filariasis, and toxocariasis • Specific studies according to focal findings (imaging studies, spinal fluid, blood smear, tissue biopsy)	To diagnose parasitic infection. It is useful to examine repeated fresh stool specimen for the diagnostics of parasite infections. Serological blood tests for schistosomiasis, filariasis, toxocariasis should be performed if the clinical suspicion is high.
• Bone marrow aspiration and biopsy • Cytogenetic analysis on bone marrow aspirate	To examine bone marrow morphology to confirm the excess of eosinophils and to exclude other haematological disorder or bone marrow infiltration. Cytogenetics on bone marrow aspirates examine the karyotype on bone marrow aspirates
• Molecular analysis on peripheral blood cells	e.g., molecular analysis for FIP1L1-PDGFRA fusion gene, molecular analysis for Wilms tumor
• Serum tryptase, serum erythropoietin, serum vitamin B12 and JAK2 mutation analysis	To diagnose myeloproliferative variant of hypereosinophilic syndrome (M-HES). Usually in M-HES and increase in serum vitamin B12 and tryptase concentration is observed
• Investigation of blood T-cells	To diagnose possible cytokine-driven eosinophilia (T-HES)
• Imaging studies (CT scan, ultrasound) of chest and abdomen	To diagnose lymphoma or non-haematological malignancy
• Serum troponin • ECG • echocardiogram	To tests for eosinophilia-mediated organ damage
• Pulmonary function tests and bronchoalvelolar lavage	To tests for eosinophilia-mediated organ damage

Adapted from: Nordic MPD Study Group. Guidelines for the diagnosis and treatment of eosinophilia. 2nd version. 2012.

The identification of organ damage is mandatory and, when present, the initiation of treatment is inevitable. It must be mentioned that the definition of eosinophilia-attributable organ involvement can represents a problem as histological evidence of tissue eosinophilia is absolutely necessary for the diagnosis.

In clinical practice obtaining histological specimens is usually extremely difficult to because the involved organs are often inaccessible for biopsy or the procedures are associated with high risk of severe complications therefore the diagnosis of hypereosinophilia-related organ dysfunction is often made by the exclusion of other causes.

Ideally, there are some laboratory test that could guide towards the diagnosis but they are often very expensive and not very disposable in all centres: immunophenotyping of T cells by flow cytometry as well as molecular assays by PCR are not widely available and can be performed only in specialized laboratories [25, 26].

Principle of Treatment

When a secondary eosinophilia is diagnosed is obvious and mandatory to focus on the specific treatment for it. More challenging is the approach to the treatment of an idiopathic eosinophilia. HES patients generally require treatment, but the management of patients with severe blood hypereosinophilia without organ involvement is still debated, since there is still no consensus on when to start the treatment in these patients [3]. Literature showed that patients with severe eosinophilia can be followed up and they may remain asymptomatic for months or even years despite the long-lasting elevation of eosinophils in blood. When eosinophils count is greater than $5.0 \times 10^9/l$, a treatment with corticosteroids may be beneficial, in order to avoid end-organ damage, but the efficacy of this management is not supported by current literature data [3]. Others prefer to start the treatment with higher counts ($>30 \times 10^9/l$), but this is, again, not supported by the evidence.

Steroids have been the first choice for long time, and their use is still quite common, with the exception for those patients with myeloproliferative HES; steroids may be useful also when there is evidence of important organ damage, such as for example in the case of myocarditis or pulmonary disease. Literature data on the dosage are confounding, it seems prudent to start with a moderate to high dose and the referred usual starting dose of corticosteroid dose is ½-1 mg prednisone/kg body weight/day. Some patients (85%) will respond to this treatment and the dose can be slowly tapered: with this approach most of the patients will respond to the therapy and moreover they will be able to be maintained on low doses for longer period [11, 12]. There are also other chemioterapic, including cytotoxic agents such a hydroxyurea which is the most extensively studied in this setting and it is associated with low side effects.

Immunomodulatory agents with effects on Th2 cytokine production and T cell proliferation can be considered useful, as for example interferon-alpha and immunoglobulin which both have been found to have significant therapeutic effects in HES, however especially with interferon-alpha important systemic side effect were reported which could actually limit its usage. Monoclonal antibody therapy, in particular monoclonal anti-IL-5 antibody therapy seems to have some advantages which are all related to the fact that IL-5 is highly specific for the eosinophils [11, 12, 27-28]. On the setting of molecular therapy a new promising but challenging horizon could be based on Sialic acid immunoglobulin- like lectins (Siglecs). Siglecs are cell surface proteins found predominantly on leukocytes. Siglec-8 is uniquely expressed on eosinophils and mast cells.

This protein is engaged in apoptosis of human eosinophils, and IL-5 priming increases Siglec-8-mediated apoptosis, a finding that may have a potential clinical implication. In fact, studies in IL-5 transgenic mice with hypereosinophilia have shown that administration of an antibody directed against Siglec-8 resulted in a prompt and significant reduction of blood eosinophilia. [29, 30, 31]

Finally, bone marrow transplantation has been used successfully in the treatment of HES, but the high morbidity and mortality of the related procedure preclude its use in most patients [3].

Conclusion

Hypereosinophilia is a clinical condition which can be potentially harmful, regardless of the possible underlying condition. Single or multiple organ damage is the principal complication which should be avoided or early detected.

Appropriate treatment is dependent in part on the ability to make an accurate causative diagnosis and to judge the clinical need for introducing an eosinophil-decreasing agent, among which steroids are still the first choice for idiopathic forms.

References

[1] Bousquet J, Chanez P, Lacoste JY, Barneon G, Ghavanian N, Enander I. Eosinophilic inflammation in asthma. *N. Engl. J. Med.* 1990. 323: 1033-9.

[2] Roufosse F. Weller P. Practical approach to the patient with hypereosinophilia. *J. Allergy Clin. Immunol.* 2010. 126: 39-44.

[3] Wagelie-Steffen A. Aceves S. Eosinophilic disorders in children. *Current Allergy and Asthma Reports* 2006. 6:475-482.

[4] Tefferi A, Patnaik MM, Pardanani A. Eosinophilia: secondary, clonal and idiopathic. *Br. J. Haematol.* 2006. 133(5):468-92.

[5] Chusid MJ, Dale DC, West BC, Wolff SM. The hypereosinophilic syndrome: analysis of fourteen cases with review of literature. *Medicine (Baltimore)* 1975. 54: 1-27.

[6] Simon HU, Rothenberg ME, Bochner BS. Refining the definition of hypereosinophilic syndrome. *J. Allergy Clin. Immunol.* 2010.126:45-49.

[7] Helbig G. Advances in the diagnosis and treatment of eosinophilia. *Curr. Opin. Hematol.* 2014. 21: 0-0.

[8] Ellis AK. Keith PK. Nonallergic rhinitis with epsinophilia syndrome and related disorders. *Clin. Allergy Immunol.* 2007. 19:87-100.

[9] Cottin V, Cordier JF. Eosinophilic pneumonias. *Allergy* 2005. 60: 841-57.

[10] Voss M, Allewelt M, Lode H.Chronic eosinophilic pneumonia. *Dtsch. Med. Wochenschr.* 2004. 129: 1858-60.

[11] Katzenstein AL. Diagnostic features and differential diagnosis of Churg-Strauss Syndrome in the lung. A review. *Am. J. Clin. Pathol.* 2000. 114: 767-72.

[12] Mehra S. Trehan A. Varma N. Marwaha RK. Hypereosinophilia: more then meets the eye. *J. Pediatr. Hematol. Oncol.* 2012. 34. e298-e291.

[13] Rieux-Laucat. Highly restricted human T cell repertoire in peripheral blood and tissue infiltrating lymphocites in Omenn's syndrome *J. Clinic. Investigation* 1998. 102 (2): 312-321.

[14] Jonczyk-Potoczna K. Hyper IgE Syndrome (Job syndrome, HIES)-radiological images of pulmonary complications on the basis of three cases. *Pol. J. Radiol.* 2012. 77(2): 69-72.

[15] Rothenberg ME. Eosinophilic gastrointestinal disorders (EGID). *J. Allergy Clin. Immunol.* 2003. 113: 11-28.

[16] Van Grotel M, de Hoog M, de Krijger RR, Beverloo HB, Van den Heuvel-Heibrink MM. Hypereosinophilic syndrome in children. *Leukemia Research* 2012. 36: 1249-1254.

[17] Weller PF, Bubley GJ. The idiopathic hypereosinophilic syndrome. *Blood* 1994. 83: 2759-79.

[18] Hary T Katz. Pediatric hypereosinophilic syndrome (HES) differs from adult HES. *Journal of Pediatrics* 2005. 146:134-6.

[19] Nelken RP, Stockman JA. The hypereosinophilic syndrome in association with acute lymphoblastic leukemia. *J. Pediatr.* 1976. 89: 771-3.

[20] Narayanan G, Hussain BM, Chandraleka B, Sivasanker C, Nair MK. Hypereosinophilic syndrome in acute lymphoblastic leukemia: case repor and literature review. *Acta Oncologica* 2000. 39: 241-3.

[21] Roufosse F, Cogan E, Goldman M. The hypereosinophilic syndrome revisited. *Annu. Rev. Med.* 2003. 54: 169-84.

[22] Brito-Babapulle F. The eosinophilias, including the idiopathic hypereosinophilic syndrome. *Brit. J. Haematol.* 2003. 121: 203 – 223.

[23] Nordic MPD Study Group. Guidelines for the diagnosis and treatment of eosinophilia. 2nd version 2012.

[24] Lorenzati A. IV Incontro Rete Ematologica Pediatrica Piemonte e Valle d'Aosta. 11 febbraio 2011.

[25] Klion A. et al. Approaches to the treatment of hypereosinophilic syndromes: a workshop summary report. *J. Allergy Clin. Immunol.* 2006. 117: 1292-302.

[26] Klion A. Hypereosinophilic Syndrome: Current Approach to Diagnosis and Treatment. *Annu. Rev. Med.* 2009. 60:293-309.

[27] Klion AD, Law MA, Noel P, Haverty TP, Nutman TB. Safety and efficacy of the monoclonal anti-interleukin 5 antibody, SCH55700, in the treatment of patients with the hypereosinophilic syndrome. *Blood* 2004. 103:2939-41.

[28] Kim YJ, Prussin C, Martin B, Law MA, Haverty TP, Nutman TB, et al. Rebound eosinophilia after treatment of hypereosinophilic syndrome and eosinophilic gastroenteritis with monoclonal anti-IL5 antibody. *J. Allergy Clin. Immunology* 2004. 114 (6):1449-55.

[29] Ilmarinen P, Kankaanranta H, Eosinophil apoptosis as a therapeutic target in allergic asthma. *Basic Clin. Pharmacol. Toxicol.* 2014. 114(1): 109-17.

[30] Takumi Kiwamoto, Norihito Kawasaki, James C. Paulson, Bruce S. Bochner Siglec-8 as a drugable target to treat eosinophil and mast cell-associated conditions, *Pharmacology & Therapeutics* 135 2012. 327–336.

[31] Ogbogu PU, Bochner BS, Butterfield JH, Gleich GJ, Huss-Marp J, Kahn JE, Leiferman KM, Nutman TB, Pfab F, Ring J, Rothenberg ME, Roufosse F, Sajous MH, Sheikh J, Simon D, Simon HU, Stein ML, Wardlaw A, Weller PF, Klion AD. Hypereosinophilic syndrome: a multicenter, retrospective analysis of clinical characteristics and response to therapy. *J. Allergy Clin. Immunol.* 2009. 124:1319.

In: Eosinophilia
Editor: Rosanna Finlay

ISBN: 978-1-63321-355-5

Chapter 4

Synovial Fluid Eosinophilia and Eosinophilic Arthritis: Updated Systematic Literature Review

Caritina Vázquez-Triñanes, M.D.[1]
and Bernardo Sopeña*, M.D., Ph.D.[2]

[1]Thrombosis and Vasculitis Unit, Internal Medicine Service, Complexo Hospitalario Universitario of Vigo (CHUVI), Vigo, Pontevedra, Spain

[2]Internal Medicine Service, Complexo Hospitalario Universitario of Santiago de Compostela (CHUS), Santiago de Compostela, A Coruña and Faculty of Medicine, University of Santiago de Compostela, A Coruña, Spain

Abstract

Synovial fluid eosinophilia is defined as the presence of eosinophils, irrespective of quantity, in the synovial fluid. This is a rare, often unexpected, and probably underestimated finding. Secondary and idiopathic forms have been described. Idiopathic forms are those not associated with systemic or rheumatic inflammatory disease or associated

* Corresponding author: Bernardo Sopeña, MD, PhD. Internal Medicine Department, Hospital Clínico of Santiago de Compostela (A Coruña-Spain). e-mail: bsopena@gmail.com.

with chronic non-inflammatory rheumatic diseases. Idiopathic synovial fluid eosinophilia can be divided into pure or pseudoallergic forms when they occur in patients with an atopic background and/or intensely positive dermographism. Their clinical significance remains incompletely understood. An updated systematic literature review on synovial fluid eosinophilia and eosinophilic arthritis is presented here. Sixty six patients with synovial fluid eosinophilia were identified after search in MEDLINE, EMBASE and Web of Science without publication date restrictions, 31 secondary forms and 35 idiopathic forms, of which 22 were pure idiopathic and 13 were pseudoallergic. Both idiopathic forms are usually monoarthritis of the large joints with a substantial component of joint effusion but few inflammatory signs. Most patients have a benign course with prompt resolution and few relapses. Non-steroidal anti-inflammatory drugs are usually sufficient to control symptoms. Peripheral eosinophilia is a rare association and is not usually severe. Synovial fluid eosinophilia, both secondary and idiopathic, has not been associated with the development of new joint deformities nor has it been described as a chronic form of arthritis.

Introduction

Synovial fluid eosinophilia is uncommon in daily practice and usually an unexpected finding. Thus, interpreting this fact may be challenging for the physician when faced with this situation. The complexity in determining the clinical significance of synovial fluid eosinophilia may be explaining by a variety of factors. First, less than 100 patients with synovial fluid eosinophilia have been reported worldwide, most of them without clinical follow-up. Second, there is no agreement on the definition of synovial fluid eosinophilia as some authors define it as the presence of eosinophils in synovial fluid (in any percentage) [1-3]; some only consider those synovial fluids with a differential count > 2% eosinophils [4]; and others when the eosinophils are present in a percentage >10% [5]. Thus, many patients with synovial fluid eosinophilia have not been studied so that the prevalence and clinical significance of the minor forms [4] (those with <10% eosinophils in synovial fluid) are poorly understood. Finally, terminological confusion exists, as some patients with peripheral eosinophilia and arthritis have been classified as having "eosinophilic arthritis" without having had an arthrocentesis, and when this procedure was performed, these patients did not present synovial fluid eosinophilia [6], while the same term have been used by other authors to denote synovial fluid eosinophilia [1, 2, 5, 7-13].

Nevertheless, although the synovial fluid is a dialysed of plasma, most authors agree that the presence of eosinophils in synovial fluid is not merely the expression of eosinophilia in peripheral blood [1, 3, 8]. For example, Idiopathic Hypereosinophilic Syndrome, Eosinophilic Granulomatosis with Polyangiitis (formerly known as Churg-Strauss syndrome), Drug Reaction with Eosinophilia and Systemic Symptoms and other conditions that occur with intense peripheral eosinophilia do not usually cause arthritis, and when they do, they do not necessarily include synovial fluid eosinophilia [6, 14-20]. On the other hand, the majority of patients with synovial fluid eosinophilia described in the literature do not have peripheral eosinophilia [1, 3, 5, 7].

To attempt to assess the clinical significance of the presence of eosinophils in synovial fluid, an updated systematic literature review on this topic was performed. So, epidemiology, aetiology, pathogenesis, clinical manifestations, diagnosis, treatment and prognosis of synovial fluid eosinophilia are discussed here.

Terms and Definitions

Synovial fluid eosinophilia is defined as the presence of eosinophils in the synovial fluid, regardless of their number and percentage [1-3, 21]. The terms "eosinophilic synovitis" and "eosinophilic arthritis" have also been used to refer to this condition [1, 2, 5, 7-13]. On this review, these terms will be avoided for reasons of terminological confusion given above.

Since the work of Brown et al. [5], synovial fluid eosinophilia is divided into two categories (major and minor forms) according to the percentage of eosinophils in the synovial fluid cell count: *minor-synovial fluid eosinophilia* when the percentage of eosinophils was <10% of total leukocytes and *major-synovial fluid eosinophilia* when the percentage of eosinophils was > 10%. This classification, later accepted by other authors [9, 22], is based on the assumption that the minor-synovial fluid eosinophilia is more common than major-synovial fluid eosinophilia and has no clinical relevance. However, this categorization is not supported by prospective studies. Although in the early works minor-synovial fluid eosinophilia was more frequent than major-synovial fluid eosinophilia [23], this has not been confirmed in any of the subsequently published series [1, 3, 7]. In addition, synovial fluid eosinophilia is dynamic and often transient, since the number of eosinophils in the synovial fluid varies over a few hours, sometimes disappearing within a few days, as evidenced with serial arthrocentesis performing [1, 4, 10, 24]. Therefore, the timing of arthrocentesis may alter the classification of the synovial fluid eosinophilia into minor or major form without thereby changes in the clinical significance. Even in recurrences of idiopathic synovial fluid eosinophilia (see below for definition and explanation), the percentage of eosinophils in synovial fluid in each episode can be so variable as to alter the classification into minor- or major-synovial fluid eosinophilia in the same patient, without apparent influence on clinical evolution and prognosis [1]. However, the fact is that in recent years the minor-synovial fluid eosinophilia have been systematically excluded from some series [5] and the vast majority of case report on synovial fluid eosinophilia, so its true prevalence and clinical significance are actually unknown.

Idiopathic synovial fluid eosinophilia was defined as those not associated with a systemic or rheumatic inflammatory disease or associated with a prior known chronic non-inflammatory rheumatic disease (like osteoarthritis) [5]. As previously reported [1, 3, 9], synovial fluid eosinophilia is classified as idiopathic when, after a careful clinical and laboratory evaluation, including complete blood cell count; erythrocyte sedimentation rate; blood chemistry profile; serum levels of IgG, IgA, IgM and IgE; antinuclear autoantibodies; nephelometric assays of C3 and C4, microbiology studies on blood and stool samples for parasites; serology for hepatitis B virus and hepatitis C virus; syphilis and anti-streptolisyn O, a known rheumatic or systemic pathology was excluded. Idiopathic synovial fluid eosinophilia is divided into *pure idiopathic and pseudo-allergic synovial fluid eosinophilia.* Pseudo-allergic synovial fluid eosinophilia occurs in patients with atopic background and / or intensely positive dermographism, as originally described by Brown et al. [5]. *Dermographism* (also called dermatographism, urticaria facticia or dermographic urticaria) is defined as the development of a wheal and flare reaction with a rapid onset after firm stroking, scratching, or the application of pressure to the skin. There are two basic forms of dermographism: simple dermographism is the more common disorder, with a prevalence from 2% to 5% in the healthy population, in which raised urticarial welts form on the skin with scratching or other stroking, but the skin is not pruritic; in symptomatic dermographism, a less common disorder, the affected skin shows urticarial welts and is pruritic [25]. In simple dermographism, the wheal typically appears within 6 to 7 minutes and begins to fade 15 to 30 minutes later; symptomatic dermographism is only slightly different, with lesions appearing in less than 5 minutes and lasting 30 minutes [26]. For the diagnosis of symptomatic dermographism, the smooth blunt object should be held perpendicular to and used to apply a light stroking pressure to the skin of the upper back or volar forearm. The skin at the test site should be unbroken and free of obvious signs of infection. If a dermographometer is available, three parallel lines (up to 10 cm long) should be made with dermographometer settings equivalent to 20, 36 and 60 g/mm^2. The reaction is considered positive in patients off antihistamines who show a weal response and report pruritus at the site of provocation at 36 g/ mm^2 (353 kPa) or less. A weal response without itch on provocation at 60 g/ mm^2 (589 kPa) or higher indicates simple dermographism. The test response should be read 10 min after testing [25]. A pressure of 64 g/ mm^2 was used by Brown et al. in their original work [5], so both simple and symptomatic dermographism were included in the definition of pseudo-allergic synovial fluid eosinophilia.

Peripheral eosinophilia was defined as the presence of >600 eosinophils/mm^3 in venous blood [27]. It was considered to be severe when there were >5000 eosinophils/mm^3 [27].

Method

A systematic review of the literature was performed by searching through the MEDLINE (source: PubMed, 1950 to February 2014), EMBASE (1974 to February 2014) and Web of Science (1900 to February 2014) databases. The following terms were used: eosinophilia, eosinophilic, synovitis, arthritis, synovial fluid, combining as MeSH terms and text words, without language restrictions. We also checked bibliographic references of previously retrieved articles and reviews from experts on this topic. Studies were eligible when they included enough clinical data, and eosinophils in synovial fluid at any percentage were documented by arthrocentesis. Data of patients with synovial fluid eosinophilia identified in the review of the literature with regard to age, sex, number of affected joints, previous joint disease, history of previous trauma to the joint, personal or family history of atopy or allergy, dermographism were collected. Clinical characteristics of arthritis and systemic manifestations, recurrences of arthritis, treatment used for each episode and joint deformity after synovial fluid eosinophilia were collected too. Laboratory data available concerning peripheral blood and synovial liquid was also analysed: erythrocytes, leukocytes -eosinophils-, crystals, and others that may be of interest. Data were analysed using the SPSS statistical program, version 18.0. The values are displayed as average and standard deviation (S.D.), median, range and percentage for quantitative and qualitative variables respectively. The T test and chi squared are used for comparisons.

Results and Discussion

The search strategy yielded 36 papers, of which 25 were case reports and case series with a total of 83 patients. Six papers, with 17 (21%) patients, were excluded because arthrocentesis was not performed (14 patients) or patients did not have synovial fluid eosinophilia as defined (3 patients). Finally, 19 articles with 66 patients with synovial fluid eosinophilia were included [1, 3-5, 7-11, 13, 22, 24, 28-34]. See graphic 1.

The 66 patients with synovial fluid eosinophilia had a mean age of 30 years ±20,7 (range 1-77 years) and 54% were male. Only 6 (10%) patients had polyarticular arthritis: 2 with rheumatoid arthritis, 1 with Sjögren syndrome with arthritis, 1 with psoriatic arthritis and 2 with idiopathic synovial fluid eosinophilia. The affected and analyzed joint was almost always the knee except for 3 ankles (1 reflex sympathetic dystrophy, 1 filariasis and 1 idiopathic synovial fluid eosinophilia), 2 elbows (idiopathic synovial fluid eosinophilia), 1 hip (chronic myeloid leukaemia) and 1 wrist (pseudogout).

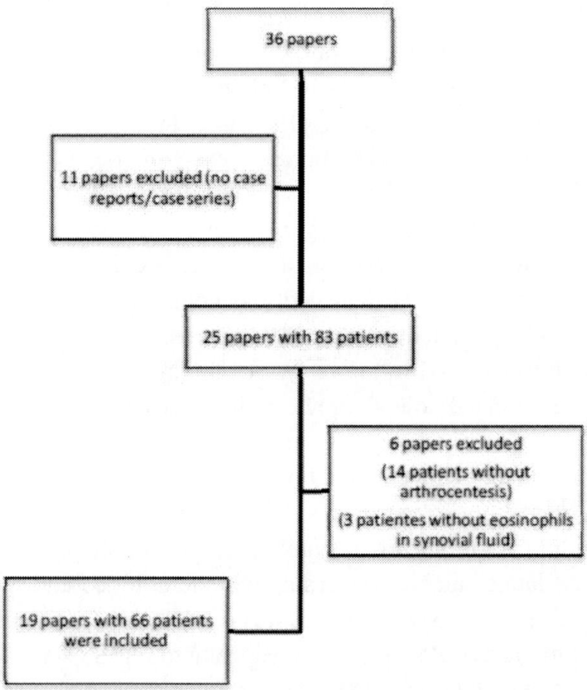

Graphic 1. Systematic literature review on synovial fluid eosinophilia and eosinophilic synovitis/arthritis process.

Table 1. Aetiology of the minor and major forms of synovial fluid eosinophilia identified in the literature review

Aetiology	n
Minor synovial fluid eosinophilia	
Hemarthrosis	3
Guinea worm	2
Chronic Myeloid	1
Leukemia Reflex sympathetic dystrophy	1
Sjögren Syndrome	1
Filariasis	1
Psoriatic arthritis	1
Major synovial fluid eosinophilia	
Pure Idiopathic	22
Pseudo-allergic	13
Post-arthrography	8
Filariasis	2
Septic arthritis	2
Lyme disease	3
Pseudogout	2
Rheumatoid arthritis	2
Psoriatic arthritis	1
Pharmacologic eosinophilia	1

Table 2. Main characteristics of pure idiopathic synovial fluid eosinophilia and pseudo-allergic synovial fluid eosinophilia published to date

	Pure Idiopathic (n 22)	Pseudo-allergic (n 13)	p
Gender, male n (%)	10 (45)	5 (38)	0,7
Mean age in years±S.D. (range)	15,7±10,37 (4-38) [if the 12 children from India published by Tauro et al. were excluded: 25±8,7 (7-38)]	30,2±16,31 (10-66)	0,01 * [0,3]
Number of affected joints	17 monoarticular, 3 oligoarticular, 2 polyarticular	12 monoarticular, 1 oligoarticular	
History of allergy or atopia n (%)	No	12 (92)	
Dermographism n (%)	No	10 (77)	
Previous trauma n (%)	1 (5)	7 (54)	0,002 *
Recurrences	32% (7/22) [if the 12 children from India published by Tauro et al. were excluded: 70% (7/10)]	38% (5/13)	0,7 [0,2]
Treatment with corticoids n (%)	2 (9)	1 (5)	0,08
Eosinophils in synovial fluid (range)	47%-90%	10%-87%	
Charcot-Leyden crystals n (%)	1(5)	4 (31)	0,05
Peripheral eosinophilia n (%)	2 (9)	2 (15)	0,06

* Statistically significant ($p<0,05$).

The literature review identified 10 patients with minor synovial fluid eosinophilia and 56 patients with major synovial fluid eosinophilia. Pathologies associated with minor and major forms are shown in table 1. Thirty one patients had secondary forms of synovial fluid eosinophilia and 35 patients had idiopathic synovial fluid eosinophilia; of which 22 were pure idiopathic and 13 were pseudoallergic. The main characteristics of patients with idiopathic synovial fluid eosinophilia are shown in table 2.

Epidemiology

Synovial fluid eosinophilia is a rare finding. In the largest series recently published, in Spain, the prevalence of synovial fluid eosinophilia was 1.02% (10 out of 982 synovial fluids) [3], slightly higher than that found in other older series from western countries. Ropes et al., in U.S., found a prevalence of synovial fluid eosinophilia of 0.86% (13 out of 1,500 synovial fluids) [23] and Amor et al., in France, 0.25% (11 out of 4,277 synovial fluids) [1]. In turn, the prevalence found by Brown et al. in Canada, was only 0.11% (13 out of 5,149 synovial fluids) [5] which may be due to the exclusion of the minor forms by these authors. Others have not found any of eosinophils in synovial fluids analyzed [35, 36]. The exception to this low prevalence is the work of Tauro et al. in India, which reports 17% [7]. Synovial fluid eosinophilia was found in 12 out of 72 synovial fluids between 1984 and 1992, all of them in children in an endemic area for filariasis. Parasites and other associated diseases were not demonstrated after a comprehensive study, so these patients were classified as idiopathic synovial fluid eosinophilia. However, a selection bias can not be ruled out in this pediatric case series. To our knowledge, there was no further work aimed to confirm this high prevalence of synovial fluid eosinophilia in this region. The presence of eosinophils and their number in synovial fluid may be underestimated in most retrospective studies and in daily clinical practice [5, 37]. This fact may be due to the degranulation of eosinophils during routine processing of the synovial liquid, which makes these cells difficult to identify [5, 37]. Brown et al. multiplied by 5 the possibility of detection of eosinophils in synovial fluid inducing the formation of Charcot-Leyden crystals (hexagonal bipyramidal structures with weakly positive birefringence under polarized light, product of the degradation of eosinophils) [5]. Some maneuvers facilitate the in vitro formation of Charcot-Leyden crystals, such as slight pressure on the cover-slip and overnight incubation at 4ºC. Detection of these crystals alerted of the possible presence of partially degranulated eosinophils that might otherwise have gone unnoticed in routine microscopic vision.

Aetiology and Pathogenesis

Synovial fluid eosinophilia has been reported in various different diseases mediated by pathogenic mechanisms that are not completely understood. Main pathologies associated with synovial fluid eosinophilia as described in the literature are shown in Table 1. Pure idiopathic synovial fluid eosinophilia and pseudo-allergic synovial fluid eosinophilia seem to be initiated by a stimulus, antigenic or mechanical. To explain the pathogenesis of pseudo-allergic synovial fluid eosinophilia, Brown et al. have proposed that the degranulation of mast cells in synovium could be due to a mechanical stimulus [5]. This explanation is based on the high frequency of dermographism and the history of a prior trauma on the joint in their case series, also reported in other studies (see table 2). The response of the synovial membrane to trauma on the joint could be similar to what occurs after the scratching over the skin with dermographism. However, as explained above, the wheal in dermographism resolved in 30 minutes but arthritis in synovial fluid eosinophilia may last several weeks. It is believed that the slower resorption of the inflammatory joint effusion may be related only to anatomic and physiologic differences between joint and skin [5]. Some authors have also questioned the relevance of simple dermographism associated with synovial fluid eosinophilia in the series of Brown et al. [37] (see section on "terms and definitions"). In fact, only one patient in their study had symptomatic dermographism [37]. It is believed that simple dermographism is an exaggerated physiological response of the skin, although its pathogenesis is incompletely understood. But simple dermographism occurs only in 5% of general population, as explained above. So, it is significant that this response of the skin was present in 10 of 35 patients with idiopathic synovial fluid eosinophilia (29%), which is a rare pathology. In the case of pure idiopathic synovial fluid eosinophilia, without dermographism per definition, a history of trauma is not so frequent (only one patient was identified in this literature review). So, a different explanation for the pathogenesis of pure idiopathic synovial fluid eosinophilia is most likely.

Whatever the nature of the stimulus that initiates the inflammatory response, mast cell degranulation seems to play a pathogenic role in the synovial fluid eosinophilia since the absence of mast cells in the synovium of patients with synovial fluid eosinophilia has been demonstrated histologically, suggesting prior degranulation of these cells [24]. That stimulus would trigger an inflammatory local response with the synthesis of Th2 cytokines, mainly IL-5, which selectively active migration and survival of eosinophils in the joint. The presence of elevated levels of IgE found in synovial fluid by some authors supports the assumption of an allergic response against an unknown antigenic stimulus [10]. This allergen bound to an IgE antibody forms a complex that binds to IgE-Fc receptors of the mast cell membrane. So this union causes degranulation of mast cells and release of eosinophilotactic substances [10]. Peripheral eosinophilia has not been reported in most of the published cases of synovial fluid eosinophilia. In the present review, only 9 patients (14%) had peripheral eosinophilia, which was severe in only one patient. This was the case of a woman with pharmacological eosinophilia and osteoarthritis of the knee where developed a synovial effusion with eosinophilia [3]. Even the frequency of peripheral eosinophilia in patients with idiopathic synovial fluid eosinophilia is similar than for patients with secondary forms (4 of 35 patients, 11%, vs 5 of 31 patients, 16%), but in any case was severe. On the other hand, Idiopathic Hypereosinophilic Syndrome, Eosinophilic Granulomatosis with Polyangiitis (formerly known as Churg-Strauss syndrome), Drug Reaction with Eosinophilia and Systemic Symptoms and other conditions that course with severe peripheral eosinophilia rarely cause arthritis and when they do, synovial fluid eosinophilia is not necessarily present [6, 14, 17, 19, 20]. Therefore, synovial fluid eosinophilia is not merely the expression of peripheral eosinophilia, although, at some point, peripheral eosinophilia may coexist with synovial fluid eosinophilia.

Only exceptionally, synovial fluid eosinophilia has been reported in patients with rheumatoid arthritis or other chronic and severe erosive arthritis [38, 39]. One possible explanation is that patients with severe erosive arthritis are often with corticosteroids or other immunomodulatory drugs in the moments of activity of the arthritis and these drugs reduce eosinophilia. Therefore, the newly developed experimental animal model is not applicable to the study of synovial fluid eosinophilia since chronic and erosive eosinophilic arthritis, not observed in clinical practice, has been induced in mice [40].

Clinical Description

Clinical manifestations of the secondary synovial fluid eosinophilia depend on the pathology associated. Systemic symptoms may accompany synovial fluid eosinophilia and may even dominate the clinical picture as in the case of septic arthritis [3], Lyme disease [4] or Sjögren syndrome [1].

Pure idiopathic synovial fluid eosinophilia and pseudo-allergic synovial fluid eosinophilia are almost always monoarthritis with large component of joint effusion, slightly painful and, usually, with few inflammatory signs. The arthritis usually resolved without specific therapy in about 7-14 days [5]. The joints most commonly affected are the knees and other large peripheral joints [1, 3, 5, 7-10, 22, 24, 28, 29]. These patients usually have no systemic manifestations. Even pseudo-allergic synovial fluid eosinophilia is not usually accompanied by symptoms of activity of allergy at the time of arthritis [1, 5, 8]. Symptomatic dermographism is actually infrequent in these patients (see section on "aetiology and pathogenesis"), so neither dermographism is a common complaint. Some patients recall having suffered trauma to the joint that may have been minimal, as explained above [1, 5, 9, 22, 24]. Difference in the frequency of a trauma to the joint as a trigger in patients with pure-idiopathic and pseudo-allergic forms has been discussed previously, in section on "epidemiology". Other features of idiopathic synovial fluid eosinophilia are shown and compared in table 2. While there may be differences in pathogenesis between pure idiopathic synovial fluid eosinophilia and pseudo-allergic synovial fluid eosinophilia, presentation and clinical manifestations of both are similar except for the trauma as a trigger, as repeatedly explained, and for the age of patients.

Although the age of patients with pure-idiopathic synovial fluid eosinophilia was lower than for pseudo-allergic form (15,7 ± 10,37 years vs 30,2 ± 16,31 years, p 0.02), a selection bias can not be ruled out. As explained in section on "epidemiology", 12 of 22 patients with pure-idiopathic form are from a pediatric case series with high prevalence of synovial fluid eosinophilia in an endemic region for filariasis [7]. If these 12 patients were excluded from the analyses, mean age of patients with pure-idiopathic synovial fluid eosinophilia were 25 ± 8, 7 years, without statistically significant difference when compared with patients with pseudo-allergic form.

Diagnosis and Diagnostic Methods

Arthrocentesis

The synovial liquid of patients with synovial fluid eosinophilia usually presents between 2,000 and 10,000 leukocytes / mm^3 although may also be less inflammatory, with 1,000-2,000 leukocytes / mm^3, as described in cases of hemarthrosis [3], post-arthrography synovial fluid eosinophilia [1] and idiopathic synovial fluid eosinophilia [1, 7, 9] and more inflammatory, even with > 10,000 leukocytes / mm^3, as in septic arthritis [3], hemarthrosis [3], pseudogout [1, 3], Lyme disease [4], filariasis [3, 7, 11], pharmacological eosinophilia [3], idiopathic synovial fluid eosinophilia [7, 24] and pseudo-allergic synovial fluid eosinophilia [8].

The percentage of eosinophils in the synovial fluid cell count probably depends critically on the time when arthrocentesis is performed rather than the specific pathology associated. This could be explained by the dynamic and transient nature of synovial fluid eosinophilia, with elevation and subsequent decrease in the percentage of eosinophils, which has been demonstrated in different studies [4, 10, 24]. As explained above, the percentage of eosinophils in synovial liquid may be even so variable as to alter the classification of synovial fluid eosinophilia in minor or major form in relapses of idiopathic synovial fluid eosinophilia in the same patient [1] with no apparent impact on the evolution and prognosis.

Charcot-Leyden crystals may be observed, but are not a common finding when routine processing of synovial fluid is performed [1, 5, 9, 30]. In the present review, these crystals were reported in 6 of the 66 patients (9%). As shown in table 2, Charcot Leyden crystals were more frequent reported in pseudo-allergic than in pure idiopathic synovial fluid eosinophilia (31% vs 5%, p 0.05). But the high prevalence of these crystals in patients with pseudo-allergic forms may be due to the inclusion of liquids in which Brown et al. routinely induced formation of Charcot Leyden crystals, as explained above.

Peripheral Blood

Peripheral eosinophilia has not been reported in most of the published cases of synovial fluid eosinophilia. In the present review, only 9 patients (14%) had peripheral eosinophilia, which was severe in only one patient. This was the case of a woman with pharmacological eosinophilia and osteoarthritis of the knee where developed a synovial effusion with eosinophilia [3]. Even the frequency of peripheral eosinophilia in patients with idiopathic synovial fluid eosinophilia is similar than for patients with secondary forms (4 of 35 patients, 11%, vs 5 of 31 patients, 16%), but in any case was severe. There was no difference in the prevalence of peripheral eosinophilia in patients with pure idiopathic and pseudo-allergic forms (table 2).

Histology

Biopsy of synovium is not necessary for diagnosis. When the synovium has been biopsied in the presence of synovial fluid eosinophilia, signs of acute synovitis, occasionally with edema and hypervascularity, and infiltration predominantly by eosinophils have been observed [1, 4, 8, 13]. Eosinophils are not always identified in synovial membrane in both secondary and pure synovial fluid eosinophilia [1, 24]. However, this fact could be influenced by the difficulty in identifying degranulated eosinophils, as explained above (section on "epidemiology"). Some authors have proposed immunofluorescence staining for major basic protein to reveal synovial eosinophilia in synovial biopsy specimens devoid of recognizable eosinophils [37], analogous to the induction of Charcot Leyden crystals in synovial fluid samples (see section on "epidemiology"). Although, to our knowledge, this procedure has never been performed.

Infiltration of the synovial membrane by eosinophils without eosinophilia in synovial fluid has also been occasionally reported, as in arthritis associated with Idiopathic Hypereosinophilic Syndrome and essential cryoglobulinemia [20, 41].

Prognosis

The presence of eosinophils in the synovial fluid has been consistently associated with a good prognosis of joint involvement. To date, no case of persistent or chronic synovial fluid eosinophilia has been described in the literature; neither synovial fluid eosinophilia has been associated with the development of new joint deformities. Recurrences are possible in idiopathic synovial fluid eosinophilia. Relapses are almost always monoarthritis, few symptomatic and self-limiting, similar with the first episode of arthritis [1, 3, 5]. There were no differences between the pure idiopathic synovial fluid eosinophilia and pseudo-allergic synovial fluid eosinophilia in terms of recurrences as shown in table 2 (32% vs 38%, no statistically significant difference). In pure idiopathic synovial fluid eosinophilia, 12 children from India with no recurrences in a short time of follow-up were included [7]. If they were excluded from the analysis, the recurrence rate would be higher in pure idiopathic synovial fluid eosinophilia (70% versus 38%, no statistically significant difference). Nevertheless, clinical significance and prognosis of pure idiopathic forms and pseudo-allergic forms seem to be similar.

Treatment

Management of secondary synovial fluid eosinophilia should be directed to the cause of arthritis whenever possible. The use of non-steroidal anti-inflammatory drugs is usually sufficient to control symptoms.

Non-steroidal anti-inflammatory drugs have been commonly used in idiopathic synovial fluid eosinophilia. Antihistaminic drugs have been occasionally used in pseudo-allergic synovial fluid eosinophilia [24]. Short course of low doses of corticosteroids has been required only in exceptional cases to control symptoms.

In the present review, 3 patients treated with corticosteroids were identified, 1 of them with pseudo-allergic and 2 of them with pure idiopathic synovial fluid eosinophilia [8, 10, 13]. The use of immunosuppressive drugs is unnecessary because of the good prognosis associated with the synovial fluid eosinophilia.

Conclusion

The frequency of synovial fluid eosinophilia is possibly underestimated in daily practice. The presence of eosinophilia in synovial fluid is associated with a benign course of arthritis.

Idiopathic and pseudo-allergic synovial fluid eosinophilia is frequently associated with self-limited arthritis, and about half of patients suffer recurrences. Non-steroidal anti-inflammatory drugs are almost always enough to control symptoms.

Unresolved Questions

The true prevalence and clinical significance of minor-synovial fluid eosinophilia are unknown, so it should not be excluded from future works.

Aetiology and pathogenesis of synovial fluid eosinophilia remain incompletely understood. Possibly, better knowledge of them may help in preventing recurrences in idiopathic and pseudo-allergic synovial fluid eosinophilia.

Competing Interests

The authors declare that they have no competing interests.

References

[1] Amor B, Benhamou CL, Dougados M, Grant A. Eosinophilic arthritis and general review of the significance of articular eosinophilia. *Rev. Rhum. Mal. Osteoartic.* 1983; 50(10):659-64.

[2] Dougados M. Synovial fluid *Baillieres Clin. Rheumatol.* 1996; 10(3):519-34.

[3] Vázquez-Triñanes C, Sopeña B, Gánzalez-González L, Díaz R, Rivera A, Freire M, Martínez-Vázquez C. Synovial fluid eosinophilia: A case series with a long follow-up. *Rheumatology* (Oxford) 2013 Feb; 52(2):346-51.

[4] Kay J, Eichenfield AH, Athreya BH, Doughty RA, Schumacher HR Jr. Synovial fluid eosinophilia in Lyme disease. *Arthritis Rheum.* 1988; 31(11): 1384-9.

[5] Brown JP, Rola-Pleszczynski M, Ménard HA. Eosinophilic synovitis *Arthritis Rheum.* 1986; 29(9):1147-51.

[6] Tay C. Eosinophilic arthritis *Rheumatology* (Oxford). 1999; 38(12): 1188-94.

[7] Tauro B. Eosinophilic synovitis *J. Bone Joint Surg. Br.* 1995; 77(4):654-6.

[8] Al-Dabbagh AI, Al-Irhayim B. Eosinophilic transient synovitis *Ann. Rheum. Dis.* 1983; 42(4):462-5.

[9] Atanes A, Fernández V, Núñez R, Galed I, Blanco FJ, García-Porrúa C, Freire M, Graña J, Galdo F. Idiopathic eosinophilic synovitis *Scand. J. Rheumatol.* 1996; 25(3): 183-5.

[10] Padeh S, Laxer RM, Gleich GJ, Armstrong PF, Silverman ED. High synovial immunoglobulin E levels in eosinophilic synovitis. *J. Pediatr.* 1992; 121(3):417-9.

[11] Kohem CL, Kristiansen SV, Kavanaugh AF. Massive eosinophilic synovitis *Ann. Rheum. Dis.* 1994; 53(4):281-2.

[12] Rayes AA, Lambertucci JR. Human toxocariasis as a possible cause of eosinophilic arthritis *Rheumatology* (Oxford). 2001; 40(1):109-10.

[13] Le Quintrec JL, Bisagni-Faure A, Gregoir C, Menkes CJ. Eosinophilic arthritis and intolerance to aspirin (Widal's syndrome). *Rev. Rhum. Mal. Osteoartic* 1991; 58:129-30.

[14] Wilkins HJ, Crane MM, Copeland K, Williams WV. Hypereosinophilic syndrome: an update. *Am. J. Hematol.* 2005; 80(2):148-57.

[15] Chusid MJ, Dale DC, West BC, Wolff SM. The hypereosinophilic syndrome

[16] Martín-Santos JM, Mulero J, Andréu JL, de Villa LF, Bernaldo-de Quirós L, Noguera E. Arthritis in idiopathic hypereosinophilic syndrome. *Arthritis Rheum.* 1988; 31(1):120-5.

[17] Baldini C, Talarico R, Della Rossa A, Bombardieri S. Clinical manifestations and treatment of Churg-Strauss syndrome. *Rheum. Dis. Clin. North Am.* 2010; 36(3):527-43.

[18] Noth I, Strek ME, Leff AR. Churg-Strauss syndrome. *Lancet.* 2003; 15; 361(9357):587-94.

[19] Cacoub P, Musette P, Descamps V, Meyer O, Speirs C, Finzi L, Roujeau JC. The DRESS syndrome: a literature review. *Am. J. Med.* 2011; 124(7): 588-97.

[20] Brogadir SP, Goldwein MI, Schumacher HR. A hypereosinophilic syndrome mimicking rheumatoid arthritis. *Am. J. Med.* 1980; 69(5):799-802.

[21] Vázquez-Triñanes C, Sopeña B. Eosinofilia sinovial. *Seminarios de la Fundación Española de Reumatología* (Revisión) 2012; 13:110-3.

[22] Amor B, Benhamou CL, Gaudouen Y, Dougados M. Eosinophilic synovitis *Arthritis Rheum.* 1987; 30(11):1313.

[23] Ropes MW, Bauer W: *Synovial Fluid Changes in Joint Disease.* Cambridge, MA, Harvard University Press, 1953, p38.

[24] Miossec P, Sullivan TJ, Tharp MD, Volant A, Le Goff P. Acute synovial fluid eosinophilia associated with delayed pressure urticaria: a role for mast cells? *J. Rheumatol.* 1987; 14(2):372-4.

[25] Magerl M, Borzova E, Giménez-Arnau A, Grattan CE, Lawlor F, Mathelier-Fusade P, et al. The definition and diagnostic testing of physical and cholinergic urticarias--EAACI/GA2LEN/EDF/UNEV consensus panel recommendations. *Allergy.* 2009 Dec; 64(12):1715-21.

[26] Kontou-Fili K, Borici-Mazi R, Kapp A, Matjevic LJ, Mitchel FB. Physical urticaria: classification and diagnostic guidelines. An EAACI position paper. *Allergy* 1997; 52:504.

[27] Tefferi A. Blood eosinophilia: a new paradigm in disease classification, diagnosis and treatment. *Mayo. Clin. Proc.* 2005; 80:75-83.

[28] Podell TE, Ault M, Sullam P, Klinenberg JR. Synovial fluid *Arthritis Rheum.* 1980; 23(9):1060-1.

[29] Luzar MJ, Friedman BM. Acute synovial fluid *J. Rheumatol.* 1982 Nov; 9(6):961-2.

[30] del Blanco J, Valverde J, Mateo L, Juanola X, Pons M, Ferrer J. Charcot Leyden crystals *J. Rheumatol.* 1991; 18(12):1944.

[31] Doury P, Saliou P, Charmot G. Eosinophilic articular effusions. Apropos of a case. *Rev. Rhum. Mal. Osteoartic.* 1984; 51(1):29-31.

[32] el Garf A. Parasitic rheumatism-Rheumatic manifestations associated with calcified guinea worm. *J. Rheumatol.* 1985; 12:976-9.

[33] Dobracki AT, Baldwing JL. A case of acute synovial fluid eosinophilia associated with delayed pressure urticaria (DPU). *J. Allergy Clin. Immunol.* 1997; 99:1369.

[34] Hasselbacher P, Schumacher HR. Synovial fluid eosinophilia following arthrography. *J. Rheumatol.* 1978; 5:173-6.

[35] Naib ZM. Cytology of synovial fluids. *Acta Cytol.* (Baltimore). 1973; 17:299-309.

[36] Lemaire V, Peltier A, Jouvent C, Ryckewaert A. Résultats de l'examen cytologique du liquid synovial dans diverses arthropathies. *Rev. Rhum. Mal. Osteoartic.* 1981; 48:229-234.

[37] Norris PG. Eosinophilic synovitis *Arthritis Rheum.* 1987; 30(10):1198-200.

[38] Tetlow LC and Woolley DE. Eosinophils are an insignificant cellular component of rheumatoid synovium in patients with a late stage disease: comparative distributions with mast cells and macrophages. *Ann. Rheum. Dis.* 1996; 55:548-551.

[39] Winchester RJ, Litwin SD, Koffler D, Kunkel HG. Observations on the eosinophilia of certain patients with rheumatoid arthritis. *Arthritis Rheum.* 1971; 14:650-665.

[40] Bockermann R, Holmdahl R. Type II collagen *Eur. J. Immunol.* 2007; 37(2):540-8.

[41] An HS, Namey TC, Kim K. Essential cryoglobulinemia associated with intense and persistent synovitis of the knee. *Clin. Orthop. Relat. Res.* 1987; 215:173-8.

Index

C

D

E

F

N

O

P

Q

R

U

V

W

X